Steve Brandl

Fascia-Puncture

Transforming Health from Within

Fascia-Puncture

Transforming Health from Within

Steve Brandl

Third Revised Edition

Imprint:

The information in this book is intended for educational purposes only. It does not constitute medical advice and is not a substitute for professional medical diagnosis, treatment, or care. The author is not responsible for any adverse effects resulting from the application of information contained herein. Always consult a qualified healthcare professional before making changes to your health practices.

Case studies in this book are drawn from clinical experience. Names and identifying details have been changed to protect patient privacy.

First published 2025

Publisher: Steve Brandl

Coverdesign: Steve Brandl

Foreword

In an era where the complexities of human health are increasingly understood through a holistic lens, the significance of fascia — our body's ubiquitous connective tissue — has finally moved into the spotlight. For too long, this intricate, interwoven matrix was largely overlooked, considered merely inert packing material around muscles and organs. The scientific community's understanding has profoundly evolved. The recent definition of fascia now recognises it as a comprehensive, uninterrupted three-dimensional web of connective tissue that extends from head to toe, front to back, and superficial to deep. It surrounds, interweaves, and interpenetrates all organs, muscles, bones, and nerve fibres. It holds our body together and enables its movements, force transmission, and communication. This living, dynamic system is not just structural but plays vital roles in immunity, inflammation, hydration, and proprioception.

Let me say plainly, early, what this book is actually about. Fascia-Puncture began as a method for working with physical restrictions in the fascial web. Over years of clinical practice, I came to see that the tissue cannot be separated from the nervous system that senses it, the predictive model that interprets it, or the personal history that shapes it. This book follows that discovery – from the fascia itself, to the mind that reads it, to the practice that works with both, to the questions neither can fully answer.

This book, Fascia-Puncture: Transforming Health from Within, delves into this profound anatomical and physiological reality, introducing a refined therapeutic approach to unlock the body's inherent healing potential. Fascia-puncture, as presented within these pages, is a precise, palpation-guided needling technique focused on releasing restrictions and restoring optimal function within this continuous fascial network. It recognises that seemingly isolated symptoms often stem from distant or hidden fascial imbalances, tracing these connections through the body's integrated fascial lines.

The importance of truly understanding fascia cannot be overstated. It is the very fabric that influences our flexibility, strength, resilience, and — as I have come to understand more deeply over the past year — even our emotional well-being and our sense of who we are. When healthy, fascia allows for fluid, effortless movement and efficient communication throughout the body. When compromised by injury, stress, or inactivity, it can become stiff, dehydrated, and adhesive, leading to chronic pain, restricted motion, and a cascade of systemic dysfunctions.

Central to the effectiveness of fascia-puncture is the cultivation of a highly refined skill of palpation. As you will discover, the practitioner's hands become the primary diagnostic tools, discerning subtle nuances in tissue tension, elasticity, and texture that guide every therapeutic intervention. This acute sensitivity enables the precise identification of dysfunctional fascial areas, leading to targeted and effective treatment.

It is worth clarifying what fascia-puncture is, and equally, what it is not. While needles are employed, fascia-puncture distinguishes itself from traditional acupuncture and dry needling in fundamental ways.

Dry needling, often performed by physical therapists or chiropractors, typically targets specific trigger points within muscle tissue, aiming to release localised muscle knots. Its focus is predominantly on muscle pain and dysfunction, often without a comprehensive appreciation of the broader fascial continuities or the more intricate physiological responses beyond a local muscle twitch.

Traditional acupuncture, rooted in ancient Chinese medicine, operates on the principles of energy meridians and qi, aiming to balance energy flow throughout the body. While it shares some superficial similarities in point locations, its underlying theory, diagnostic methods, and therapeutic goals are fundamentally different, based on a philosophical and energetic framework rather than the anatomical and physiological understanding of fascia.

Fascia-puncture, conversely, is grounded directly in the cutting-edge understanding of modern fascia research. It meticulously maps and treats the body's fascial lines and their interconnections, recognising that restrictions in one area can transmit tension and dysfunction far afield. It is a systematic, anatomically informed approach that seeks to restore the dynamic, adaptable nature of the entire fascial web, thereby catalysing profound and holistic improvements in health, movement, and overall well-being.

Since the first edition of this book was published, my understanding has deepened in ways I did not anticipate. In February 2026, I published The Storytelling Monkey and the Web of Life, a book that follows the neuroscience of the self as far as it honestly goes and then stands at the boundary where it stops. Writing that book forced me to take seriously what I had been observing in clinical work for two decades: that the fascial web is not merely a structural system that occasionally holds emotional residue. It is the primary somatic site of the stories the brain tells about who we are. The brain's Default Mode Network generates the narrative. The predictive hierarchy maintains it. And the fascia – the living, innervated, mechanically responsive matrix that runs from skull to sole – is where that narrative takes up physical residence. This understanding informs every chapter of the second edition.

This book offers a comprehensive guide for both practitioners seeking to deepen their understanding of fascial science and integrate this powerful therapeutic modality, and for anyone curious about the remarkable potential of their own body's connective tissue to transform health from within.

Disclaimer

The medical insights shared here are for informational purposes and should never replace the personalised guidance, diagnosis, or treatment provided by your healthcare practitioner.

It is critical to understand that the treatment methods described in this book, particularly those involving needling such as fascia-puncture, require specialised medical training. This book does not constitute a medical qualification and does not substitute for comprehensive professional training in acupuncture, dry needling, or any other medical procedure. Individuals considering the application of these techniques must be fully aware of and comply with all legal requirements and professional licensing regulations within their specific country or jurisdiction to ensure they are adequately trained and legally permitted to provide such treatments. Always prioritise patient safety and adhere to the highest standards of professional practice.

PART ONE

The Fascial Body

What fascia is, how it behaves, and why the body is interconnected

The clinical and anatomical foundation of Fascia-Puncture.

The Making of a Fascia-Puncturist

"Learn to move among the world without becoming trapped by praise or blame. This is called profound sameness"

– Daodejing, Chapter 56

The practitioner's intellectual history is its own version of the Storytelling Monkey's journey: from one framework to another, each one genuinely useful, each one eventually revealing its own blind spots – until the accumulated evidence of sustained palpation finally suggests that the territory has been there all along, waiting for the maps to be held lightly enough to let it be seen directly.

How I Arrived Here

I trained as a massage therapist and physical therapist in Germany, completing my qualifications in 2006. The framework I received was the standard Western one: the body as a collection of discrete, nameable structures — muscles, bones, nerves, joints, organs — each capable of developing specific, diagnosable conditions that responded to specific, evidence-based interventions. This is an extraordinarily powerful framework. I am not being ironic. The biomechanical model of the human body has produced anaesthesia, surgery, the germ theory of disease, antibiotics, joint replacements, and the reduction of infant mortality to a fraction of what it was two centuries ago. When I need emergency medicine, I want the mechanical model. I want the surgeon who knows exactly which structure is damaged and exactly how to repair it.

But the mechanical model has a blind spot that becomes impossible to ignore the moment you place your hands on a living body. The textbook shows muscles as isolated red shapes, bordered cleanly from their neighbours, attached to bones at defined origin and insertion points. The living body under the hands is not this. It is continuous. The boundaries between the structures the textbook names are, in living tissue, gradients rather than walls. The muscle does not end and the fascia begin. They are woven together in a web that does not respect the categories the textbook has drawn around them. The model was built on cadavers – tissue from which the fluid had drained, from which the tensions of living had been released, from which the three-dimensional organisation of living fascia had collapsed into the flat, separable layers that a dissection knife could distinguish. The map was drawn from dead territory. I was practising on the living.

The Second Map: Traditional Chinese Medicine

In 2013, I completed my training in Traditional Chinese Medicine. I had come to TCM because the mechanical model was not answering questions I encountered daily on the treatment table. Why did restriction in this patient's shoulder respond to work at the hip? Why did chronic thoracic pain so consistently co-present with breathing dysfunction that bore no mechanical relationship to the site of pain? Why did some patients' tissue respond rapidly under sustained, light contact, while others with apparently identical presentations showed almost no response to the same technique?

TCM offered a different map. Qi – vital energy flowing through the meridian system, disrupted by illness and restored by needling. The twelve primary meridians, the extraordinary vessels, the five elements, the patterns of organ disharmony. A framework rich in clinical observation, accumulated over millennia of careful practice, that could identify patterns and predict responses in ways the mechanical model had no language for. I was grateful for this framework. I still am. The clinical intelligence embedded in the classical Chinese medical texts is extraordinary – not because the ancient practitioners had access to modern imaging or neurophysiology, but because they were working from direct, sustained, palpation-based observation of living bodies across an enormous span of clinical time. They were, in the most important sense, empiricists.

But the map they built had, in its transmission to the contemporary clinic, become as fixed as the mechanical model it was supposed to complement. The meridians that the classical texts described as dynamic, responsive pathways, defined by clinical palpation and subject to revision, had been standardised into the printed diagrams that hang on the walls of acupuncture schools worldwide: fourteen primary channels, 361 classical points, their precise locations measured in anatomical landmarks and cun from specified reference positions. The living geography of energy flow had become a circuit diagram. The Monkey had arrived, named everything, and filed it.

This is the Monkey's relationship to every tradition it inherits: it receives a map drawn from direct experience, names the elements of the map, standardises the locations, and gradually begins to treat the chart as the territory. The original practitioners were empiricists. Their successors became cartographers. The difference is the difference between attending to what the hands find and consulting what the textbook says should be there.

Departing from the Sanctioned Map

The first time I placed a needle where my hands found the restriction rather than where the diagram specified the classical point, I felt the specific unease of a practitioner departing from the sanctioned map. I was trained to needle Stomach 36, Liver 3, Lung 7. I was needling the density and restriction my palpation found two centimetres from Stomach 36, following the actual distribution of fascial engagement rather than the printed location. The results were better. My discomfort was considerable.

This discomfort is not trivial and is worth naming. Every medical tradition generates a community of practice, and every community of practice generates its orthodoxy. The practitioner who departs from the orthodoxy is departing from the shared language of the community – the language that allows practitioners to communicate, to teach, to receive referrals, to be understood by patients who arrive with expectations shaped by that same orthodoxy. It took me several years, and a significant accumulation of clinical observation, to arrive at a framework that could justify what the hands had already been doing.

The framework, when it came, was not invented. It was already present in the research literature. Helene Langevin's work at the University of Vermont had, by the early 2000s, produced compelling evidence that acupuncture points – located by palpation in living subjects, as the classical practitioners had originally found them – consistently overlapped with points of significantly greater connective tissue density. The needle, rotated at these points, generated a measurable mechanical response in the surrounding fascia: collagen fibres winding around the needle in the tissue coupling that the classical literature called de qi – the arrival of Qi – and that the laboratory showed to be a measurable fascial engagement.

The meridians were not imaginary lines. They were, in all likelihood, patterns in the fascial web – the continuous connective tissue matrix that Guimberteau's endoscopic imaging had revealed as genuinely, uninterruptedly continuous from skull-crown to the soles of the feet. The channels the classical practitioners had mapped by palpation corresponded, with striking frequency, to the myofascial lines that Thomas Myers described in his anatomy trains model: the Superficial Back Line, the Lateral Line, the Deep Front Line, the Spiral Line – each a fascial continuity that transmits tension and force through the entire body, and each running through the approximate territory of one or more classical meridian channels.

This was not a vindication of classical TCM as literal description. The qi that flows through the meridians is not a substance that can be measured. The five elements are a metaphorical system of correspondences that has clinical utility without having biological literalness. What the research suggested was something more precise and more interesting: that the ancient practitioners, working from palpation of living tissue over millennia, had found and mapped the fascial web before the fascial web had been named. Their map was not a fantasy. It was a map drawn in a different language, by people attending to the same territory through a different window.

Fascia-Puncture: Neither Map

What I was doing – following the palpatory signal rather than the textbook location, needling the fascial restriction rather than the printed point – was not a departure from the spirit of the classical tradition. It was, arguably, a return to it. The earliest acupuncture was palpation-based. The standardisation that produced the printed charts came later, driven by the need for a teachable, transmissible protocol that did not depend entirely on the practitioner's accumulated tactile intelligence. The protocol was useful. It was also a map drawn at one remove from the territory.

Over the years that followed my TCM training, the two frameworks I had been working with – the mechanical model of Western physical therapy and the energetic model of TCM – began to be replaced by something that was neither and both. Not a synthesis – I am suspicious of syntheses, which tend to inherit the blind spots of both parents and the advantages of neither. Something more like a return to the territory that both frameworks had been trying to map: the living fascial web, the continuous, fluid, mechanically responsive, neurologically dense connective tissue matrix that the body actually is, as distinct from both the discrete-structure model and the energy-channel model that the two traditions had overlaid on top of it.

The approach I gradually developed I came to call Fascia-Puncture – a term I chose carefully and want to be equally careful to explain. It is palpation-guided needling of the fascial web. Not acupuncture as TCM defines it – I am not treating Qi or balancing organ disharmonies according to five-element theory. But not dry needling as the Western physiotherapy model defines it either – I am not needling trigger points in isolated muscles according to the mechanical model. I am following what palpation finds in the three-dimensional continuity of the fascial web, and I am working with the tissue's own intelligence – its viscoelastic responsiveness, its capacity to rehydrate and reorganise under sustained, gentle mechanical stimulus – rather than imposing a protocol on top of it.

I explain this to new patients who arrive expecting classical acupuncture: the needle, in my practice, is not a key that unlocks energy flow at a classical point. It is a precision instrument for mechanical intervention in the fascial web. Its rotation engages the collagen fibres of the connective tissue, generating a mechanical signal that propagates through the web and stimulates the mechanoreceptors embedded in the fascia, which communicate with the central nervous system and can change the autonomic tone and the predictive model the brain is running about the state of that tissue. This is not mystical. It is biomechanics at the scale of connective tissue fibres. Some patients find this clarification disappointing. They came for Qi. Most, I have found, are curious rather than disappointed – and those who are curious tend to engage most fully with the work, because they are already holding their map of the body lightly enough to be surprised by the territory.

A word about what Qi means to me now, because I do not want to be misread as dismissing it. Qi, as a concept, is one of the most elegant clinical metaphors in the history of medicine. The idea that living systems have a quality of vital animation – dynamic, flowing, directional, distinguishable from mechanical force – is not primitive superstition. It is an attempt to name something genuinely real: the aliveness of living tissue, its capacity for self-organisation, its responsiveness to attention and to change. When I feel the difference between tissue that is vital and responsive and tissue that has withdrawn into dense, dehydrated immobility, I am feeling what the classical practitioners called deficient Qi. The name is different. The palpatory reality is the same. What I reject is not the concept but the fixing of it. Qi that is alive and useful is Qi that flows – discernible only through palpation of the living tissue, not through reference to a chart. Qi that becomes a cage is Qi frozen into a printed diagram, its locations standardised, its practitioner's task reduced to inserting needles at the correct GPS coordinates rather than following the tissue's actual report.

The Drop of Knowledge

A phrase I have been using with students for several years is at the centre of what I am attempting with Fascia-Puncture and with this book.

Accumulated knowledge in any field – but particularly in medicine – does something specific to the practitioner who accumulates it. It trains the perceptual system to find what the training has prepared it to find. The Western-trained physical therapist palpates a shoulder and finds the discrete structures the anatomy textbook has named: supraspinatus, infraspinatus, subscapularis, joint capsule, bursae. The TCM-trained acupuncturist palpates the same shoulder and finds the flow qualities of the Small Intestine and Triple Warmer channels, the De Qi response at SI 11 and TW 15, the excess or deficiency pattern the tongue and pulse have already suggested. Both practitioners are genuinely feeling something real. Both are filtering the felt reality through a framework that makes some things visible and others invisible.

Palpatory wisdom is what becomes possible when you set both frameworks down – not permanently, not dismissively, but in the way the Daodejing recommends setting down the map when you want to see the territory directly. It is the accumulated, embodied intelligence that has passed through both frameworks and come out the other side — not as a synthesis of the two but as a quality of attention that can use either framework as a tool without being contained by either as a cage. I call it the drop of knowledge not because the knowledge is discarded — it is not. The years of training in anatomy, in clinical reasoning, in the classical Chinese medical literature are present in every session. They are present the way musical theory is present in a skilled improviser's playing: structuring what is possible, available when needed, not crowding out the direct response to what is actually happening. The drop is more like a breath out. A deliberate softening of the grip that formal knowledge tends to maintain on perception. An act of not-knowing that makes room for the tissue's actual report.

The Daodejing expresses this in Chapter 48: in pursuit of learning, something is acquired daily. In pursuit of the Dao, something is dropped daily. What is dropped, in the practice of palpatory wisdom, is not the learning but the learning's insistence on being right. The insistence that the restriction must be at Stomach 36 rather than two centimetres lateral. That the presenting symptom must match the textbook. That what the hands are finding must be explicable within the available framework, rather than evidence that the framework needs expanding. I have been practising this dropping for twenty years. I am not yet very good at it. The Monkey is always present, always ready to classify, to name, to fit the unfamiliar sensation into a known category. But the practice of attending to what the hands actually find – before the trained practitioner in me has had a chance to file it – has produced, session by session, a clinical intelligence that neither of my training frameworks fully prepared me for. It is the intelligence of the tissue itself, accessed through a quality of attention that the tissue apparently rewards with disclosure.

What Remains to Be Learned

A closing note that I find both honest and, unexpectedly, encouraging. I do not know if

Fascia-Puncture is a mature approach. I am not certain it is even a stable one. The framework I am working within – palpation-guided needling of the fascial web, understood through the lens of connective tissue mechanics, predictive processing, and EMFT – is not a finished system. It is where I currently am in a process that began when I noticed, in my first year of clinical practice, that the tissue under my hands was telling me something the textbook had not prepared me for.

The research on fascial mechanics is advancing faster than clinical practice can currently absorb. Guimberteau's endoscopic imaging keeps revealing new levels of structural organisation in living connective tissue that the dissection table never showed. The neuroscience of interoception and predictive processing keeps producing findings that reframe what the tissue's mechanoreceptors are actually doing when a needle engages the collagen fibres. The clinical research on pain reprocessing therapy and somatic approaches keeps providing evidence for mechanisms that clinical observation had been pointing at for decades before the trials confirmed them.

What I practise now may look, in ten years, the way what I practised in 2010 looks to me now: a genuine but preliminary attempt, shaped by the knowledge and tools available at the time, correct in its direction but limited in its depth. This possibility does not trouble me. It is the condition of any honest practice. The practitioner who is certain they have arrived is the practitioner who has stopped attending. Laozi describes the sage as someone who, having walked far, still does not consider the destination reached. Not because the destination recedes — but because the quality of attention that genuine practice produces makes the territory continuously richer, continuously more surprising, continuously more capable of teaching. The tissue has been teaching me for twenty years. I expect it will teach me for twenty more. The question I bring to the treatment table has not changed: what is actually here, before I name it? The answer has never been the same twice.

What the body knew:

Neither map was wrong. The mechanical model showed me what the tissue was made of. The energetic model showed me how the tissue moved. What neither map could show me was the tissue itself — the living, continuous, fluid, narratively intelligent web that both maps were trying to describe. The hands found it directly, when the maps were held lightly enough to let it be seen. What the body knew was never contained in either tradition. It was in the territory they were both pointing at.

What My Hands Found

Before the anatomy, before the mechanism, before any of the science that fills the chapters ahead — a case. This is the kind of thing my hands found, early in the practice this book describes, that the standard maps could not explain.

Mr. A presented with a chief complaint of debilitating migraines, predominantly localised to the left side of his head, though rarely affecting the right. The painful area typically originated in the lateral neck and occipital region, radiating around the ear and extending to a few centimetres above the left eye. These excruciating episodes, occurring approximately once a month, were frequently accompanied by nausea and severe light sensitivity, with little or no precursory aura. His medical history was otherwise unremarkable, with no significant injuries or surgeries; however, he reported occasional sleep disturbances and increased stress due to a demanding work schedule. While certain alcoholic beverages could sometimes trigger these migraines, most occurrences were unpredictable. Despite these debilitating headaches, Mr. A maintained an otherwise healthy lifestyle, consistently preparing home-cooked meals and integrating daily cycling into his commute.

Initial palpation provided critical insights, revealing significant fascial restrictions. On the left side, particularly, pronounced tightness was noted in the lateral and medial lines of the neck and occipital areas. This tension ascended to involve the temporal and parietal fascial layers and also descended into the lateral shoulder and anterior medial clavicle-sternum region. Adhering to the principle of fascial interconnectedness, palpation extended to include the distal arm and leg areas. Restrictions were identified in the lateral and posterior arm lines, and the anterior, lateral, and medial lines of the lower legs.

Our tailored healthcare plan commenced with two fascia-puncture sessions per week for five weeks, followed by a maintenance phase of one session per week for an additional five weeks. On average, each session involved the precise placement of approximately 45 needles in a face-up position. Typically, 20 to 25 needles were strategically positioned on the left head, neck, and shoulder area, directly addressing the palpated restrictions. When needling the anterior neck region, exceptional caution is paramount due to the presence of vital structures such as the carotid arteries, major nerves, and the thyroid gland. An additional 10 to 15 needles were placed on the contralateral right head, neck, and shoulder regions. The legs received 3 to 4 needles per side, and the arms usually 2 per side. For the lower legs and arms, traditional acupuncture points often served as an initial orientation, around which meticulous palpation was performed within a few centimetres to determine the optimal precise location and angle for needle insertion.

From the first session, Mr. A reported gradual and consistent improvements. Remarkably, he experienced zero excruciating migraines since the commencement of treatments, only mentioning two instances of manageable, far less severe dehydration headaches. This case illustrates how the systematic application of the body's simplified fascial divisions can yield profoundly appropriate clinical outcomes.

The Body's First Whispers

An Embryonic Journey into Our Inner Landscape

Think back to the very beginning – not your first memory, but a time before you even had a body as you know it. It all started with a single cell, a microscopic universe brimming with potential. This was not just any cell; it held the complete instruction manual for creating you, a unique and intricate being. This chapter is not about complex biology jargon; it is a story of incredible transformation, a glimpse into the astonishing choreography that turns one tiny spark into the magnificent machine that is the human body. We will follow the early stages, meet the key players, and marvel at the forces that shape us from the very first moments of existence. From this seemingly simple beginning arises the intricate architecture of the human body, a framework interwoven with a remarkable network of connective tissues.

Our story begins with a dramatic encounter: fertilisation. A sperm, a tiny vessel of genetic information driven by an ancient urge, embarks on an epic journey to find its counterpart, the egg. The egg, a relatively large and patient cell, awaits this crucial meeting. When a single, determined sperm successfully penetrates the egg's outer layer, it triggers an immediate and profound change. The egg's surface alters, preventing any other suitors from entering, and the precious cargo of genetic material from both sperm and egg merges. This fusion creates the zygote, the very first cell of a new individual, containing a complete set of instructions – your original blueprint. This newly formed zygote, now containing the complete genetic code, immediately embarks on its first crucial step of development: cellular division.

The zygote does not simply grow bigger; instead, it initiates a series of rapid-fire cell divisions called cleavage. Imagine a master baker quickly dividing a lump of dough, again and again, creating smaller and smaller portions. The zygote divides into two cells, then four, then eight, and so on, forming a solid ball of cells known as the morula. Each of these early cells, called blastomeres, holds a complete copy of the original blueprint. This rapid multiplication of cells is not chaotic; it is a highly organised preparation for the next stage, where these cells will begin to differentiate and form a more complex structure.

The morula then undergoes a fascinating reorganisation, transforming into a structure called the blastocyst. This is a hollow sphere with two distinct groups of cells, each with a vital role. The outer layer of cells, the trophoblast, will eventually develop into the placenta, the incredible organ that will nourish and sustain the developing embryo, acting as a crucial lifeline connecting the growing life to the mother. Inside this sphere is the inner cell mass, a cluster of cells holding the promise of the future embryo – the source from which all the tissues and organs of the body will arise. This small group of cells is where our focus sharpens.

Now comes a period of intense activity and organisation called gastrulation. The relatively simple ball of cells undergoes a dramatic rearrangement, forming three distinct layers, like a skilled artist carefully layering different colours onto a canvas to create a complex image. These layers are the primary germ layers, the fundamental building blocks of the entire body.

Imagine the outermost layer, the ectoderm, as the body's surface and its communication network. It will give rise to the skin, our protective barrier and sensory interface with the world. Even more remarkably, it forms the entire nervous system, including the brain, the intricate control centre, and the spinal cord, the main communication highway. Our senses – sight, hearing, smell, taste, and touch – all have their origins in this outer layer.

The middle layer, the mesoderm, is the body's construction crew, responsible for building our framework and our ability to move. It will develop into muscles, the engines of our motion; bones, the supportive scaffolding; blood, the vital fluid that nourishes and cleanses; the heart, the tireless pump that drives this flow; and, crucially for our later exploration, the connective tissues, which include the extensive network of fascia.

The innermost layer, the endoderm, will form the linings of our internal systems, the tubes and surfaces that allow us to breathe and digest. It will give rise to the lining of the digestive tract, from the mouth to the intestines, as well as the lungs, the organs of respiration, and other vital organs like the liver and pancreas.

Gastrulation is a pivotal moment, establishing the fundamental architecture of the body, setting the stage for the incredible specialisation and organisation that will follow. These three primary germ layers are not just temporary structures; they are the foundational blueprints that will give rise to every tissue and organ in the body.

Let us take a closer look at the mesoderm's incredible versatility. This middle layer is not just one type of tissue; it is a dynamic source of a wide array of crucial components that make us who we are. From the tiny muscles that allow our eyes to blink to the large muscles that propel us through space, the mesoderm provides the building blocks for all our voluntary and involuntary movements. The bones that give us structure, support, and protection all arise from the mesoderm. The heart, the tireless organ that pumps life-giving blood throughout our bodies, and the intricate network of blood vessels that carry oxygen and nutrients to every cell, all originate from the mesoderm.

The connective tissues are the body's glue and network – this is where our focus on fascia truly begins. The mesoderm gives rise to all the connective tissues, including tendons that connect muscle to bone, ligaments that connect bone to bone, cartilage that provides cushioning, and, most importantly, fascia, the continuous web that surrounds and permeates all these structures, as well as muscles and organs.

The early embryo starts as a relatively flat disc, but it does not remain that way for long. A remarkable and precisely orchestrated process called embryonic folding transforms this two-dimensional structure into the complex three-dimensional form of the human body. This folding is driven by differences in growth rates and coordinated movements within the three germ layers. The mesoderm plays a crucial role in this shaping process, contributing to the formation of the body cavities and the precise positioning of our internal organs.

As the embryo folds, spaces begin to form within its structure – the future body cavities. The thoracic cavity will house the heart and lungs, protected by the rib cage. The abdominal cavity, below the diaphragm, will contain the digestive organs, liver, kidneys, and other vital structures. The pelvic cavity will house the bladder, reproductive organs, and the lower part of the digestive tract. The mesoderm lines these cavities with specialised membranes, providing support and reducing friction as organs move.

Even as the mesoderm contributes to the overall shaping of the embryo, it is also diligently constructing one of the first functional organs: the heart. A simple tube of mesodermal cells begins to form and, incredibly, starts to beat spontaneously. This tiny, rhythmic pulse is one of the earliest signs of life, a testament to the powerful drive for development and the intricate instructions encoded within our very first cell. This early heartbeat establishes the flow of nutrients and oxygen that will fuel further growth and differentiation.

While the mesoderm is busy shaping the physical structure and the circulatory system, the ectoderm is undergoing its own remarkable transformation, laying the foundation for our nervous system. A groove forms along the back of the embryo, a crucial step in neural tube development. This tube will eventually close and differentiate into the brain, our complex control centre, and the spinal cord, the main communication pathway between the brain and the rest of the body. This early wiring is the beginning of our ability to sense, move, and think.

Around this time, small swellings known as limb buds begin to appear on the sides of the developing embryo. The mesoderm within these buds will proliferate and differentiate to form the bones, muscles, and connective tissues – including fascia – that will make up our arms and legs, allowing us to reach, grasp, walk, and interact with the world around us.

None of this intricate development happens by chance. A complex symphony of signals guides it. Genes turn on and off in specific sequences, dictating which cells will become which tissues. Cells communicate with each other through a variety of chemical signals, influencing their neighbours' behaviour. Even physical forces play a role, guiding the shape and organisation of developing tissues. It is a dynamic and interactive process of incredible precision.

Morphogens are powerful signalling molecules that diffuse from specific cells and create concentration gradients, essentially acting as positional cues. Cells respond to different concentrations by activating different genes, leading to cell differentiation and tissue patterning. Growth factors are a broader category of signalling molecules that stimulate cell growth, proliferation, and differentiation. Cell adhesion molecules on the cell surface help cells stick together and to the extracellular matrix, playing a vital role in tissue organisation. The extracellular matrix itself influences cell behaviour by interacting with cell surface receptors and storing signalling molecules. The extracellular matrix is a crucial part of fascial tissues.

This intricate dance of signalling molecules ensures the precise development and organisation of all tissues, including the body-wide tensional network of fascia. Fascia is considered a body-wide tensional force transmission system. Cellular communication is key to how mechanical forces are translated into biological responses within tissues, a process called mechanotransduction.

In the delicate dance of embryological development, timing is absolutely critical. Each stage must occur in the correct sequence and at the appropriate pace. Even slight disruptions can have significant consequences. As we have journeyed through these early stages, we have seen the mesoderm as the origin of so many vital tissues, including the connective tissues. Among these, fascia stands out as a continuous and pervasive network that will eventually permeate the entire body. In later chapters, we will delve deeply into the remarkable properties and functions of fascia – how it supports our structure, facilitates movement, plays a role in sensory perception, and even influences our emotional landscape. But understanding its embryological roots in the mesoderm highlights its fundamental and unifying role in our very being.

From a single, microscopic cell, a complex and beautifully organised human being emerges. This incredible journey, guided by the genetic blueprint within the zygote and orchestrated by the dynamic interactions of the three primary germ layers, is a testament to the power and elegance of life itself. The story of embryology is not just a scientific explanation of how we are formed; it is a profound reminder of the intricate and miraculous beginnings of each and every one of us. And woven through it all, from the earliest mesoderm onward, runs the thread that this book follows: the living web of fascia.

Nourishing the Lord of Life

Excerpt from Chapter 3 of the Zhuangzi

Lord Wenhui was watching his cook carve up an ox. The cook's hands moved with a whir, his shoulders with a lurch, his feet stamped, and his knees bent – with a hiss! with a thud! – the flesh came apart as the knife sang, every movement in perfect rhythm, like the dance of the Mulberry Grove, or the chords of the Jing Shou.

"Ah, excellent!" cried Lord Wenhui. "How did you attain such skill?"

"What your servant values is the Dao, which goes beyond mere skill. When I first began to carve oxen, all I saw was the ox itself. After three years, I no longer saw the whole form, but rather the intricate structure within. And now, I move with my spirit rather than my eyes. My senses stop functioning and my spirit moves as it wills, intuitively navigating the natural spaces of the ox as I glide the knife through the great crevices and along the natural openings, never touching the slightest ligament or tendon, much less a large bone."

"A good cook changes his knife once a year because he cuts – he hacks. An average cook changes his knife once a month because he nicks – he chips. But this knife of mine has been used for nineteen years and has carved thousands of oxen, yet its blade is as sharp as if it had just come from the whetstone."

"This is because I move it through the spaces. Where there are joints, there are spaces, and the blade of my knife finds ample room. There is no congestion, no obstruction. That is why my knife remains as good as new."

"Of course, when I come to a complicated place, I see the difficulty and become cautious. My eyes focus, my movements slow, and I wield the knife with the utmost care. Then, with a subtle movement – wham! – the flesh parts like earth crumbling. Then I lift my knife and stand up, look all around, and with satisfied deliberation, wipe my knife clean and put it away."

Lord Wenhui exclaimed, "Excellent! From the words of this cook, I have learned how to nourish life!"

This insightful passage is from chapter 3 of the Zhuangzi (4th–3rd century BCE), a foundational Daoist text. Cook Ding's mastery of the spaces within the ox, allowing his knife effortless movement, mirrors how a practitioner can sense and work with the inherent spaces within the fascial network.

The text highlights something of profound clinical relevance: that ancient practitioners focused on physical tissue spaces rather than unseen energy pathways. The knife does not cut through the ox; it follows the ox's own architecture. In the same way, the practitioner's hands – and eventually the needle – do not force the tissue; they follow where the tissue leads.

There is a quality of attention in Cook Ding's work that I recognise in the best moments of clinical practice. It is the attention that arrives when the practitioner has moved beyond mere technique into something closer to participation. The tissue speaks; the hands listen; the intervention follows the architecture that is already there. The neuroscience of flow states – the reduction in prefrontal self-monitoring, the quieting of the Default Mode Network – describes this condition precisely. The Monkey steps back, and what remains is direct engagement with what is present. This is not mysticism. It is a description of the organism functioning at its actual capacity, without the interference of its own narrative commentary.

The Anatomy and Physiology of Fascia

The Unseen Architecture of You

Step into the intricate and often overlooked world of fascia, the body's pervasive connective tissue network. Imagine a scaffolding that not only holds every part of you together, from the deepest organs to the outermost layers of skin, but also actively influences how you move, feel, and function as a whole. Understanding this unseen architecture is fundamental, especially for appreciating the profound impact of therapies like fascia-puncture, which interact with this very system to promote healing and well-being throughout the entire body.

Imagine peeling an orange. The white, fibrous web that clings to the fruit and segments its juicy interior – that is a glimpse into the world of fascia, albeit a simplified one. Now, amplify that image across your entire body: a continuous, three-dimensional network of connective tissue that is far more intricate and vital than mere packing material. This unseen architecture, this fascial web, permeates everything, from the tips of your toes to the crown of your head, with the intriguing exception of the open passageways of your lungs and digestive tract – those hollow tubes rely on their own specialised linings and structures.

For years, fascia was often relegated to the sidelines of anatomical study, viewed as the stuff you had to cut through to get to the "important" bits – the muscles, bones, and organs. But a revolution in understanding is underway, revealing fascia as a dynamic, active tissue with a multitude of crucial roles. Think of it as the body's internal tailor, constantly surrounding, supporting, separating individual structures, and, most importantly, connecting them all into a functional whole. It divides muscle groups, allowing for coordinated action, and ultimately contributes to the very shape and functionality of your physical form.

Forget the idea of isolated muscles or organs. Fascia creates a breathtakingly continuous network throughout your entire being. Imagine a silken thread woven through every layer, connecting your tendons, your joint capsules, and even the delicate envelopes surrounding each muscle. This interconnectedness means that a seemingly small restriction in one area can have ripple effects throughout the entire system – a tight band in your calf might influence the way your shoulder moves, for instance. In The Storytelling Monkey and the Web of Life, I describe this as the Web of Life – not as metaphor but as anatomical fact. The fascia is the physical substrate of the body's unity.

Your body is constantly adapting to the stresses and strains you place upon it, and fascia is a key player in this remarkable ability. Think of it as a living fabric that adjusts its weave and tension based on your history of movement and load. A dancer's fascia will adapt differently to the demands of ballet than a weightlifter's will to heavy lifting. This adaptability is crucial for resilience and efficient movement, but it also means that prolonged periods of inactivity or repetitive strain can lead to less optimal fascial architecture. And, as we will explore later, the fascia adapts not only to physical forces but to emotional ones as well – to the sustained tensions of chronic stress, suppressed anger, unresolved grief. The tissue records the life lived in it.

If you were to explore the fascial system, you would discover it is not a single sheet but rather a complex layering, each with its own characteristics and roles.

The first layer lies immediately beneath your skin. This superficial fascia is more than just a cushion; it allows your skin to glide smoothly over deeper tissues, enabling a wide range of movement without pulling or restriction. It also houses nerves, blood vessels, and lymphatic channels, making it a crucial interface with the external world and a key player in fluid dynamics.

Beneath the superficial fascia lies the deep fascia, a denser and more organised layer of connective tissue that invests the musculoskeletal system. This layer plays a critical role in compartmentalising muscles, facilitating their function, and providing structural support. In some areas, deep fascia takes the form of aponeuroses – broad, flat sheets of tendon-like tissue that serve as attachments for muscles. These aponeuroses, such as the lumbar fascia, are also part of the deep fascial network and play a crucial role in transmitting forces and stabilising the spine.

Within the dynamic world of movement, the fascia associated with our musculoskeletal system takes on a particularly crucial role, often referred to as myofascia. This is not just about a superficial wrapping; it is an intricate and inseparable partnership where muscle and connective tissue are interwoven at every level, acting as the very language through which our bodies express motion.

Think of a single muscle. What appears to be a homogenous unit is, in fact, a highly organised collection of individual muscle cells, also known as muscle fibres. Each of these slender fibres, the fundamental contractile unit of muscle, is itself enveloped by a delicate layer of fascia called the endomysium. This endomysium provides structural support to each individual muscle fibre, ensuring that the force generated during contraction is effectively transmitted along the length of the fibre. It also carries the tiny blood vessels and nerves that nourish and activate each muscle cell.

These individual muscle fibres do not work in isolation. They are organised into bundles called fascicles. Each fascicle is surrounded by another layer of fascia, the perimysium. This layer is thicker and more robust than the endomysium, providing further structural integrity to the muscle by grouping these fibres together. The perimysium also contains larger blood vessels and nerves that supply the fascicles.

Finally, the entire muscle itself is encased by a dense outer layer of fascia known as the epimysium. This is the most superficial layer of the myofascia, providing a strong and cohesive outer boundary for the entire muscle belly. But here is where the interconnectedness becomes truly fascinating: the endomysium, perimysium, and epimysium are not separate, distinct layers that abruptly end at the muscle. Instead, they are continuous with the connective tissues that extend beyond the muscle itself to form tendons – the tough, fibrous cords that anchor muscles to bones.

The collagen fibres that make up the endomysium coalesce and become organised into the collagen fibres of the perimysium, which in turn contribute to the collagenous structure of the epimysium. As the muscle transitions into a tendon, these continuous fascial layers become even more densely packed and aligned, forming the incredibly strong and resilient tissue that can withstand the immense forces generated by muscle contraction.

Therefore, the "myo" and "fascia" are not truly separate entities but rather different expressions of the same continuous connective tissue matrix. This seamless integration ensures that the force generated by the contraction of individual muscle fibres is efficiently transmitted through the fascial network, across the muscle belly, and ultimately to the bone via the tendon, creating movement. This perspective truly highlights how muscles do not act as isolated motors pulling on levers. Instead, they function as specialised contractile units embedded within a vast and interconnected fascial sleeve. Understanding this intimate relationship is key to appreciating how fascial restrictions within the muscle itself can impede movement and how releasing these restrictions can have a profound impact on overall function.

Just as your muscles and bones are enwrapped by the intricate layers of somatic fascia, so too are your internal organs invested by visceral fascia. This fascial layer provides crucial support, suspends organs within the body cavities, and, as you move, allows them to glide smoothly against one another, preventing friction and entanglement. Imagine your intestines, constantly shifting and turning during digestion – it is the visceral fascia that facilitates this dynamic movement without causing chaos within your abdomen.

The role of visceral fascia extends beyond simply supporting and allowing movement of the organs themselves. This fascial network also intimately surrounds and organises the vital pathways that supply and innervate these organs: the blood vessels and the nerves. Arteries and veins are carefully encased in layers of fascia that provide structural support, protect them from external pressures, and help anchor them within the surrounding tissues. This fascial wrapping ensures that these delicate vessels maintain their integrity and patency, allowing for the unimpeded flow of blood.

Similarly, your nervous system extends throughout your viscera, controlling their function and relaying sensory information back to the brain. Just like muscles, these nerves are not simply single strands; they are complex structures composed of individual nerve fibres bundled together. Fascia plays a key role in organising these neural pathways. Individual nerve fibres are surrounded by a delicate layer of connective tissue. These fibres are then grouped into bundles, or fascicles, which are encased by a more substantial layer of fascia. Finally, the entire nerve trunk is surrounded by an outermost layer of connective tissue. This fascial organisation within nerves serves structural support, organises the bundles, provides vascular supply through small blood vessels, and offers protection from compression.

Therefore, visceral fascia is not just about the organs themselves; it is also about the intricate organisation and support of the blood vessels that feed them and the nerves that control them. This highlights the pervasive and essential role of fascia in maintaining the overall health and function of our internal world, ensuring that everything is not only supported but also properly connected and supplied.

The Fundamental Components

Collagen, Elastin, Ground Substance, and Cells

Fascia, this remarkable connective tissue, is not just a uniform substance but a dynamic composite material. To truly appreciate its function, we need to explore its fundamental building blocks.

Collagen is the primary fibrous protein that provides fascia with its tensile strength, its ability to resist being pulled apart. However, it is not a one-size-fits-all molecule; there are many different types of collagen, each with a specialised role. Type I Collagen is the most abundant type in the body and the primary collagen of tendons, ligaments, and deep fascia. It is incredibly strong and forms thick fibres that are highly resistant to stretch. Type III Collagen is often found alongside Type I; this collagen is more prevalent in the skin and blood vessels. It is thinner and contributes to tissue elasticity. Other types like Type IV and Type V also play important roles in specific fascial structures, while Types I and III are dominant in most fascia.

The arrangement of collagen fibres within fascia is crucial for its function. In tendons, collagen fibres are densely packed and aligned longitudinally, like the fibres in a rope, to withstand the high tensile loads generated by muscle contractions. In other areas, such as the superficial fascia, collagen fibres may be arranged in a more multi-directional or irregular weave, providing flexibility and allowing for movement in various directions. Collagen is not static; it constantly adapts to mechanical demands. Fibroblasts, the cells responsible for collagen synthesis, respond to tension and stress by altering the production and organisation of collagen fibres, a process that is key to tissue remodelling.

While collagen provides strength, elastin fibres provide elasticity, the ability of fascia to stretch and recoil. Elastin fibres are interwoven with collagen fibres, allowing fascia to deform under load and then return to its original shape. This elasticity is particularly important in areas where movement and flexibility are essential, contributing to the body's ability to store and release energy during locomotion.

Surrounding the collagen and elastin fibres is the extracellular matrix, a complex and dynamic gel-like substance that is far from being inert. The primary component of the ECM is the ground substance, a hydrated gel that fills the spaces between cells and fibres. Glycosaminoglycans are a key component of the ground substance. These are long, unbranched polysaccharides that attract and bind water. Hyaluronic acid is a prominent GAG in fascia, contributing to its viscosity and lubrication. The ground substance is rich in water and ions, creating a fluid environment essential for nutrient and waste exchange, for cellular communication through the diffusion of signalling molecules, and for providing a medium for mechanical forces to be transmitted. The state of water in the ECM is important; in healthy fascia, a significant portion exists as "bound water," exhibiting liquid crystal-like behaviour. This unique state contributes to fascia's ability to glide and adapt.

Proteoglycans are large molecules consisting of a core protein attached to GAGs. Proteoglycans contribute to the ECM's structure and hydration. Understanding this fluid environment is key to appreciating how various therapeutic approaches can influence tissue health.

The primary cells within fascia are fibroblasts. Fibroblasts are responsible for synthesising and maintaining the ECM, including collagen, elastin, and the ground substance. Fibroblasts are not passive; they are highly sensitive to mechanical stimuli, such as tension, compression, and shear forces. This process, known as mechanotransduction, allows fibroblasts to sense the mechanical environment and respond by altering their gene expression and metabolic activity. For example, increased tension can stimulate fibroblasts to produce more collagen, leading to tissue strengthening. Through mechanotransduction, fibroblasts play a crucial role in the continuous remodelling of fascia, adapting its structure and composition to the body's needs.

How Fascia Senses and Responds

The Power of Mechanotransduction

This detailed exploration reveals that fascia is far more complex than simple wrapping. It is a dynamic tissue whose properties arise from the intricate interplay of diverse components, all working together to provide support, facilitate movement, and respond to the forces of life. This ability of fascia to respond to mechanical stimuli is a fundamental principle underlying many manual therapies.

Perhaps one of the most groundbreaking revelations about fascia is its crucial role in transmitting mechanical forces throughout the body. Your muscles do not work in isolation, pulling directly on bones; they often act in concert with the fascial network to create efficient and coordinated movement.

Fascia links groups of muscles together, forming what are known as myofascial slings. Think of these slings as integrated chains that work together during complex movements like walking, running, or throwing. For example, a sling involving muscles in your back and opposite hip helps to stabilise your pelvis during locomotion. Understanding these slings is crucial for analysing movement patterns and addressing imbalances.

In specific regions, like the lumbopelvic area, fascia plays a critical role in transferring loads. The thick, multi-layered lumbar fascia acts as a bridge between muscles and bones, helping to stabilise the spine and distribute forces during bending, lifting, and twisting. Its health and integrity are paramount to prevent back pain.

Thomas Myers' groundbreaking concept of Anatomy Trains, or myofascial meridians, offers a powerful framework for understanding the body's interconnectedness beyond individual muscles. These Trains are not simply lines drawn on a diagram; they represent real, functional continuities within the fascial web, describing how muscles and fascia collaborate to distribute forces, maintain posture, and create movement.

Instead of viewing muscles as isolated units, Myers proposes that they are organised into long, continuous lines of myofascia, much like train lines connect different cities. Tension or restriction in one station along the line can create imbalances and dysfunction in other, seemingly distant stations. This perspective helps explain why a tight calf muscle might contribute to lower back pain or why restricted movement in the shoulder can affect hip mobility.

The Superficial Back Line runs from the plantar fascia under the foot, up the back of the legs, along the back, and over the skull to the forehead. It primarily functions to support the body in an upright position and to facilitate extension movements. Restrictions can contribute to plantar fasciitis, hamstring tightness, and back pain.

The Superficial Front Line runs from the top of the foot, up the front of the legs, across the front of the torso, and up the neck to the skull. It is involved in flexion movements and provides a counterbalance to the SBL. Tightness here can pull the body into a flexed posture, contributing to rounded shoulders and breathing restrictions.

The Lateral Line travels along the sides of the body, from the foot and ankle, up the lateral leg, along the torso, and up the neck. It plays a key role in lateral stability and balance. Imbalances can contribute to lateral trunk flexion and hip issues.

The Spiral Line wraps around the body in a double spiral, connecting the foot, lateral leg, back, shoulder, and neck. It is crucial for rotational movements and maintaining balance during complex activities.

The Arm Lines connect the arms to the torso and are subdivided into Deep and Superficial Front and Back Arm Lines. They are essential for arm movement, shoulder function, and posture.

The Functional Lines are engaged during specific activities, such as walking or throwing, and connect the shoulder to the opposite hip. They are crucial for coordinated movement patterns and power transfer.

The Deep Front Line is considered one of the most central and influential myofascial meridians in the body. Unlike the more superficial lines, the DFL is a complex, multi-layered continuum that runs deep within the torso, connecting the arches of the feet to the top of the head. It traverses the inner aspects of the legs, ascends through the pelvis, continues through the front of the spine, the rib cage, and finally reaches the neck and skull. The Deep Front Line is crucial for core stability, postural support, and efficient movement. Restrictions within it can have far-reaching effects on posture, breathing, organ function, and movement patterns throughout the entire body.

The Anatomy Trains concept has significant clinical implications. By mapping these myofascial connections, practitioners can identify the root cause of pain rather than just treating the site of pain, develop holistic treatment strategies, improve movement efficiency, and enhance postural alignment.

Building upon this understanding of force transmission, it is essential to acknowledge the significant contributions of Luigi Stecco and his Fascial Manipulation method. Stecco's work provides another influential perspective on how the fascial network organises and transmits forces. Stecco developed a comprehensive biomechanical model that emphasises the role of fascia in musculoskeletal pain and movement limitations. His approach centres on myofascial units – functional units composed of muscles, their associated fascia, and the articular surfaces they influence. Stecco proposed that these units are interconnected through specific directional vectors within the fascial planes.

Stecco identified specific fascial sequences running through the body in six primary directions. A key element of his model is the identification of Centres of Coordination and Centres of Fusion – areas where forces from different directional sequences converge and integrate. Palpation and treatment of these specific points are central to the Fascial Manipulation technique, aiming to restore proper tension and glide within the fascial planes.

There are striking similarities between the acupuncture meridians and the myofascial meridians of Thomas Myers, and the fascial sequences of Luigi Stecco. While Traditional Chinese Medicine often describes acupuncture meridians as channels for vital energy, a closer look at ancient texts like the Zhuangzi suggests that ancient practitioners also focused on the physical, tangible pathways within the body, such as tissue planes and natural openings. When you compare anatomical charts of these different systems, you will notice that they often follow comparable routes through the body. The naming and interpretation might differ – one system emphasising energy flow, another emphasising force transmission – but the underlying pathways share significant commonalities. They might all be mapping the same underlying anatomical structures, primarily the connective tissue network.

The Mechanics of Movement

Fascia's Dynamic Role

Furthermore, fascia's influence extends beyond the musculoskeletal system to other systems in remarkable ways. The thoracolumbar fascia connects muscles of the trunk, abdomen, and pelvis, playing a crucial role in core stability and force transfer during movement. Fascial connections also influence breathing mechanics, as the diaphragm is connected to surrounding fascial structures. These connections highlight the interconnectedness of the body and how fascial tension in one area can affect the function of distant regions, demonstrating the body-wide communication facilitated by the fascial network.

In the field of sports and movement, healthy and adaptable fascia is crucial for athletic performance, movement efficiency, and injury prevention. The elastic recoil of fascia enhances power and reduces energy expenditure during dynamic movements. Optimal fascial glide allows for smoother, more coordinated movements, improving performance and reducing the risk of injury.

To address fascial health and dysfunction, various therapeutic approaches directly target the fascial system. These include manual therapies such as massage and myofascial release, movement therapies such as yoga, pilates, and qigong, and needling techniques including acupuncture, dry needling, and fascia-puncture. By addressing fascial restrictions, promoting healthy tissue glide, and restoring optimal fascial tension, these interventions can reduce pain, improve movement, and enhance overall well-being.

Moving beyond its anatomical structure, we delve into the fascinating and increasingly appreciated physiology of fascia. It is not merely a passive wrapping or container for our muscles and organs; rather, it is an active and dynamic participant in how our bodies move, stabilise, sense the world around us and within us, and even communicate on a cellular level. A key aspect of this dynamic role lies in fascia's unique mechanical properties.

Imagine the fascial network as a pre-loaded, body-wide tensional system, a continuous web maintaining a baseline level of tension throughout the body. This inherent tension, often referred to as pre-tension or tone, is not static but rather a dynamic readiness to respond to forces. This pre-tension provides a supportive framework for all movement, allowing for efficient force transmission from muscles to bones and distributing forces throughout the body. When a muscle contracts, it pulls on this pre-tensed fascial network, and the resulting change in tension is propagated throughout the system, contributing to the overall movement and stability of the body. This interconnectedness means that muscle action is never truly isolated; it always occurs within the context of this fascial web.

Adding to this dynamic interplay, fascial tissues, particularly those with a higher proportion of elastin fibres, exhibit significant elasticity, enabling them to store and release mechanical energy. Think of the Achilles tendon during running: as the foot lands, the tendon is stretched, storing energy; during push-off, this stored energy is released, contributing to propulsion and reducing the metabolic cost of locomotion. This elastic recoil is crucial for efficient and dynamic movements, including walking, running, jumping, and throwing, allowing for a spring-like action that enhances power and reduces the energy expenditure required by muscles. This storage and release of energy is not limited to tendons; it occurs throughout the fascial network, contributing to the fluidity and efficiency of movement.

Beyond this elastic response, fascia also demonstrates viscoelasticity, a property that lies between pure elasticity and pure viscosity. This means that its mechanical behaviour is influenced by both the rate and duration of the applied force. When a force is applied rapidly, fascia behaves more like an elastic solid, resisting deformation. However, when a sustained force is applied, fascia exhibits a more fluid-like behaviour, gradually yielding and lengthening. This characteristic explains why slow, sustained stretches are more effective in increasing fascial length and flexibility compared to quick, ballistic movements. Viscoelasticity allows fascia to adapt to sustained postures and repetitive movements over time, contributing to both stability and adaptability.

Fascia is not just a structural tissue; it is also a richly innervated sensory organ, playing a vital role in proprioception, kinesthesia, and interoception. The fascial network is densely populated with various mechanoreceptors, specialised nerve endings that respond to mechanical stimuli. These receptors are sensitive to a wide range of stimuli, including stretch, pressure, vibration, and shear forces. These mechanoreceptors constantly transmit information to the central nervous system, providing crucial feedback about the state of the musculoskeletal system. Manual therapies, movement therapies, and needling techniques can effectively stimulate these mechanoreceptors, influencing pain perception, muscle tone, and proprioceptive awareness.

This rich sensory input is fundamental to our body awareness. Proprioception is the body's sense of its position and orientation in space, even without visual input. Fascia plays a critical role by providing a rich source of sensory information about muscle length, tension, joint position, and movement. Kinesthesia, closely related to proprioception, is the sense of movement, allowing us to perceive the speed, direction, and amplitude of our movements. The fascial contribution to proprioception is so significant that damage or dysfunction to fascia can lead to impaired movement coordination and balance.

There is an additional dimension to the sensory capacity of fascia that deserves attention. The neuroscientist Anil Seth has proposed that the brain is fundamentally a prediction machine — continuously generating its best model of what is happening inside and outside the body, then comparing that model against incoming sensory data. Fascia, as one of the body's most richly innervated tissues, feeds an enormous amount of sensory information into this predictive system. When fascial restrictions alter the quality or volume of proprioceptive and interoceptive signals, the brain's model of the body changes. The restriction does not merely limit movement; it alters the organism's sense of itself. This is why patients sometimes describe the resolution of a long-held restriction not merely as the absence of pain but as feeling like a different person. The self-model has updated.

Furthermore, fascia has intricate connections with other systems, contributing to their function and integration. The thoracolumbar fascia connects muscles of the trunk, abdomen, and pelvis, playing a crucial role in core stability and force transfer during movement. Fascial connections also influence breathing mechanics, as the diaphragm is connected to surrounding fascial structures. These connections highlight the interconnectedness of the body and how fascial tension in one area can affect the function of distant regions.

The richness of receptors in fascia plays a significant role in sensitivity to weather changes, a phenomenon known as meteoropathy. Fascia is densely populated with mechanoreceptors sensitive to pressure. Changes in atmospheric pressure can exert pressure on our tissues, including fascia, triggering these receptors and sending signals to the nervous system. Individuals with scars, recent recoveries, or old injuries may experience heightened sensitivity. Temperature changes can also affect fascial tissues directly. Cold temperatures can cause tissues to contract, while heat can lead to expansion, further stimulating mechanoreceptors.

Fascia also plays a vital role in internal communication, coordinating cellular activity and tissue responses. This communication occurs through cellular crosstalk, where fibroblasts are highly responsive to mechanical signals through mechanotransduction. Fibroblasts sense mechanical forces through various receptors and transform these forces into biochemical signals, triggering intracellular changes. This regulates the production and remodelling of the extracellular matrix, allowing fascia to adapt to mechanical demands.

Furthermore, fascia plays a role in a subtle feedback loop involving muscle spindles. Intramuscular fascia interacts closely with muscle spindles, sensory receptors that detect changes in muscle length and the rate of change. The condition of the intramuscular fascia can influence the sensitivity and firing rate of muscle spindles, affecting proprioception, muscle tone, and motor control. Fascial restrictions can alter muscle spindle function, potentially contributing to movement impairments and pain.

Fascia is a dynamic and adaptable system that constantly remodels itself in response to mechanical demands. Regular and specific movements can stimulate fibroblasts to realign collagen fibres, alter the density and thickness of fascia, and improve its elasticity and glide. Conversely, prolonged inactivity, immobilisation, or repetitive strain can lead to fascial thickening, stiffening, and the formation of adhesions. However, while fascia is adaptable, its turnover rate is generally slower than that of muscle tissue. Changes occur gradually and require consistent effort. Allowing 36 to 48 hours between heavy physical activity sessions is generally advised for adequate recovery.

A deeper understanding of fascial anatomy and physiology has significant implications for various clinical fields. Fascial restrictions, adhesions, and altered tension are increasingly recognised as major contributors to musculoskeletal pain and movement disorders. Healthy and adaptable fascia is crucial for athletic performance, movement efficiency, and injury prevention. Various therapeutic approaches directly target the fascial system, including manual therapies, movement therapies, and needling techniques. By addressing fascial restrictions, promoting healthy tissue glide, and restoring optimal fascial tension, these interventions can reduce pain, improve movement, and enhance overall well-being.

In conclusion, fascia is more than just a wrapping tissue. It is a dynamic, sensory, and communicative network that plays a vital role in every aspect of our movement, stability, and overall health.

The Pathophysiology of Fascia

When Fascia Fails to Glide

Just like any complex system, the fascial network is susceptible to dysfunction. Various factors can lead to changes in its structure and properties, resulting in pain, restricted movement, and other discomforts. Understanding these pathological changes is crucial for appreciating the rationale behind interventions like fascia-puncture.

One key aspect of fascial dysfunction involves changes in collagen and elastin. Trauma, inflammation, and even prolonged immobility can disrupt the delicate balance of these fibres within the fascia. Collagen fibres, which provide tensile strength, may become excessively cross-linked, leading to stiffness and reduced elasticity. Simultaneously, elastin fibres, responsible for recoil, might lose their ability to snap back, further contributing to restricted movement.

The ground substance, the gel-like matrix that lubricates fascial layers, is also critical for healthy movement. Dehydration, often due to insufficient water intake or chronic inflammation, can cause this ground substance to become viscous and thickened. This increased viscosity hinders the smooth gliding of fascial planes, leading to feelings of stiffness and a restricted range of motion. A helpful analogy is to think of a sponge: a dehydrated sponge is brittle and resists movement, much like dehydrated fascia.

Increased fascial tension and the development of trigger points are other common manifestations of dysfunction. Physical or emotional stress can lead to sustained muscle contractions, which in turn can increase tension within the surrounding fascia. Over time, these areas of increased tension can develop into trigger points – hyperirritable spots within a taut band of muscle that can refer pain to other areas of the body. The fascia surrounding these trigger points often becomes thickened and restricted, perpetuating the problem.

The body's healing processes can also contribute to fascial dysfunction. Following injury or surgery, the body initiates a repair process that involves the deposition of collagen fibres to mend damaged tissues. While essential for repair, excessive or disorganised collagen deposition can lead to the formation of adhesions – abnormal connections between fascial layers that restrict movement and can cause pain. Scar tissue, a denser form of collagen, can also limit flexibility and alter the mechanical properties of fascia.

Inflammation, whether acute or chronic, has a direct impact on fascia. Inflammatory mediators can sensitise the nerve endings within the fascia, leading to increased pain perception.

Furthermore, prolonged inflammation can contribute to structural changes within the fascia, creating a self-sustaining cycle of pain and dysfunction.

Finally, and crucially for this second edition, it is important to acknowledge the role of Emotional Myofascial Tensions – what I call EMFT. This concept, which was briefly introduced in the first edition, has since become central to my clinical understanding. Repressed emotions can manifest as chronic muscle contractions and fascial tension. This sustained tension contributes to the pathological changes described above, further restricting movement and amplifying pain signals. In my clinical model, the fascia does not merely record physical events; it appears to record something of the emotional climate in which those events occurred. A shoulder injury sustained during a period of intense personal conflict may heal differently – and hold a different quality of restriction – than the same injury sustained during a period of relative calm. The tissue remembers more than anatomy alone can explain. I will return to this subject at length in the chapter devoted to it.

Cultivating a Healthy Fascia Web

General Practices

It is worth emphasising the importance of Vitamin D for fascial health. Adequate levels of vitamin D are believed to support fascial integrity and flexibility, helping to prevent stiffness and dysfunction. Many people, particularly those in northern climates or who spend significant time indoors, may not get sufficient vitamin D through sunlight alone. Consider having your levels checked and supplementing if necessary.

Beyond specific nutrients, the overall quality of your diet matters. Processed foods, refined sugars, and inflammatory vegetable oils – those high in Omega-6 fatty acids – contribute to a systemic inflammatory state. This continuous inflammation promotes the breakdown of connective tissue, encourages stiffening, and hinders the body's ability to utilise water effectively, leaving the ECM dehydrated and prone to restriction. Therefore, avoiding foods rich in sugar is a foundational step in reducing systemic inflammation and promoting fascial fluidity.

The balance between activity and rest deserves further attention. Fascia thrives on movement, but both overuse and underuse can lead to problems. Aim for a varied exercise routine that incorporates different types of movement. This helps ensure that all parts of the fascia are being used and not overstressed. Allowing 36 to 48 hours between heavy physical activity sessions is generally advised for adequate muscle and connective tissue recovery. This time frame allows muscles to repair and rebuild, reducing the risk of injury and improving performance.

Maintaining a healthy fascia web involves a multifaceted approach that encompasses nutrition, balanced activity, and specific exercises. This chapter outlines general practices to promote fascial health, focusing on accessible and sustainable strategies.

Just as a balanced diet is crucial for overall well-being, it also plays a significant role in fascial health. Key nutrients support fascia's structure, hydration, and ability to repair and remodel.

Hydration is paramount. Fascia contains a significant amount of water, which is essential for its flexibility and lubrication. Dehydration can lead to stiff, sticky fascia, restricting movement and increasing the risk of pain. Aim for adequate daily water intake. Anti-inflammatory foods are equally important. Chronic inflammation can negatively impact fascia, contributing to pain and stiffness. An anti-inflammatory diet rich in omega-3 fatty acids, antioxidants, and whole, unprocessed foods can help reduce inflammation and support tissue health. Collagen support through nutrients like Vitamin C, amino acids, and copper is essential for collagen synthesis. Adequate levels of vitamin D are believed to support fascial integrity and flexibility.

The balance of activity is critical – avoiding both overuse and underuse. A sedentary lifestyle leads to fascial stiffening, thickening, and the formation of adhesions. Regular movement is crucial to keep fascia hydrated, flexible, and healthy. Even standing up and moving around for a few minutes each hour can make a difference. Repetitive movements can strain certain areas, causing tightness and potentially leading to adhesions. Varying activities and ensuring proper form are important to prevent overuse injuries. Aim for a varied exercise routine that incorporates different types of movement.

Walking is a simple yet effective way to promote overall fascial health. It improves circulation, which is vital for fascia hydration and flexibility. A daily brisk walk for 20 minutes can have an amazing impact on health and well-being. This does not mean we have to run marathons.

Jumping, whether with or without a rope, strengthens lower leg muscles and improves the elasticity of the surrounding tendons and fascia. It also improves coordination and balance, contributing to overall body awareness.

Gentle stretching – regular, slow, sustained stretches – is crucial for maintaining fascial flexibility and range of motion. It helps release tension, improve blood flow, and promote relaxation. Focus on techniques that release tension in the connective tissue rather than simply pulling at muscles.

By incorporating these principles into daily life, it is possible to cultivate a healthy and resilient fascia web, supporting pain-free movement, optimal performance, and overall well-being.

Imaginary Jump Rope - A Fascial Exercise

By following these guidelines, imaginary jump rope can be a highly beneficial and safe exercise to enhance the vitality and resilience of your entire fascial web. The key is consistency and listening to your body. Start gently, progress gradually, and always prioritise soft, controlled landings. Over time, you will notice improvements in your balance, coordination, and the overall springiness of your movement – all signs of a healthier, more responsive fascial system.

It is worth noting that jumping exercises can be particularly beneficial for the elastic component of fascia. Research has shown that the fascial system responds especially well to bouncing, springy movements that engage its elastic recoil capacity. By regularly practising imaginary jump rope, you are training not just your muscles but your entire fascial network to become more efficient at storing and releasing elastic energy – the very mechanism that makes movement feel effortless and light.

Imaginary jump rope, also known as shadow jumping or air jumping, is a fantastic way to engage your fascial system, improve cardiovascular health, and enhance coordination without needing a physical rope. It is a low-impact exercise that can be done almost anywhere. Here is how to do it properly and what to watch out for to prevent injury.

Wear supportive athletic shoes that provide good cushioning and absorb impact. Avoid jumping barefoot on hard surfaces, as this can stress your joints and fascia. If you want to jump barefoot, do it on softer surfaces or outdoors. Choose a forgiving surface – a mat, a sprung floor, or grass is ideal. Avoid concrete or asphalt.

Before you start, perform a gentle warm-up. This could include light marching in place, arm circles, leg swings, and some dynamic stretches like ankle rotations. This prepares your muscles and fascia for activity.

Stand tall with your feet hip-width apart, knees slightly bent. Your gaze should be forward, and your shoulders relaxed, not hunched. Hold your hands as if you are gripping a jump rope, close to your body. Rotate your wrists in small, quick circles, mimicking the motion of turning a rope.

The movement should primarily come from your wrists, not your entire arms.

The jump should be small and controlled. Push off the balls of your feet, keeping your knees slightly bent to absorb impact. Land softly on the balls of your feet, allowing your heels to gently touch the ground afterward. Find a steady, rhythmic bounce. Coordinate your wrist rotation with your jumps.

The beauty of imaginary jump rope for fascia is the ability to vary the movements, which loads the fascial system in different ways. Two-foot bounces – both feet lift and land together, focusing on a springy, elastic bounce. Alternating feet in a running-in-place style introduces more shear and rotational forces through the fascial lines. High knees and butt kicks increase the range of motion and dynamic stretch on the fascial chains. Single-leg jumps enhance balance and put more localised load on the fascial structures of that leg. Side-to-side jumps engage the lateral fascial lines. Small rotations with each jump activate the spiral fascial lines.

Start slowly and gradually increase. If you are new to jumping, begin with short intervals – 30 seconds jumping, 30 seconds rest – and gradually increase as your stamina and fascial resilience improve. Focus on soft landings. This is critical. Landing softly on the balls of your feet with slightly bent knees allows your fascia and joints to absorb impact efficiently. Maintain good posture. Slouching can put unnecessary strain on your neck and back fascia. Monitor for pain. Any sharp, sudden, or persistent pain is a signal to stop. Stay hydrated. Incorporate gentle stretching and a cool-down after your jumping session. Vary your routine by incorporating other activities like walking, gentle strength training, and mobility work.

Practical Guidance - For Optimal Health and Well-being

Making daily movement a habit is fundamental. Opt for the stairs instead of the elevator whenever possible. Incorporate brisk walks into your morning or evening routine. Even 15 to 30 minutes can make a significant difference. Engage in gentle cardio exercise – cycling, using an elliptical, or rope jumping – 3 to 4 times per week. These activities are excellent for cardiovascular health without excessive strain.

Supporting the Fascial Environment

Fascia is not immune to what you eat. Ground substance needs hydration to stay fluid; collagen synthesis needs vitamin C, zinc, and adequate protein; and systemic inflammation – driven largely by highly processed foods, excess sugar, and oxidised oils – stiffens the very matrix this book is about. You do not need a rigid system to act on this. Favour whole, minimally processed foods; keep processed meats, fried foods, and sugar-heavy products occasional rather than routine; and drink enough water that your tissue has something to work with. That is the whole principle. The unique contribution of this book is not nutritional advice – it is what follows.

Functional Breathing - Light, Slow, Deep, and Nasal Breathing

Of everything in this chapter, the single most powerful daily practice is breath. I use a simple framework for it: LSD – Light, Slow, Deep, always through the nose. Light means minimal force, almost silent. Slow means roughly six breaths a minute – five seconds in, five seconds out. Deep means directed into the belly, not the chest. Practised for ten minutes, twice a day, this alone measurably shifts the nervous system from threat to safety, and safety is where fascia softens. Part III returns to this practice in full depth – the vagus nerve, the science of why it works, and the complete 5:5 protocol – because by then you will also understand the Monkey it is quieting.

The Internal Work - Qigong and the Mastery of Breath-Energy

Should you wish to deepen your practice of Qigong, there are many forms to explore – from the gentle flowing movements of Ba Duan Jin, the Eight Pieces of Brocade, to more complex forms involving standing meditation and martial applications. Each has its own value. But the foundation remains the same: the breath, the tongue position, and the quality of awareness you bring to whatever you happen to be doing at this moment. The practice is always available, because the breath is always available.

In my own practice, I have found that the moments of greatest clinical insight – the moments when the hands seem to know what the tissue needs before the mind has formed a theory about it – coincide with the moments of deepest breathing rhythm. The hands become more sensitive when the breath is slow. The needle finds its place more naturally when the practitioner is not rushing. The patient's nervous system settles more readily in the presence of a practitioner who is themselves settled. This is not a coincidence. The co-regulation of nervous systems through shared breathing rhythm is a well-documented phenomenon in polyvagal research. Your own breath, as a practitioner, is as much a part of the treatment as the needles you use.

Beyond specific routines, the true value of Qigong lies in its underlying philosophy: the mastery of internal energy through conscious breath. This concept offers a profound framework for integrating the principles of Light,

The same Light, Slow, Deep principle simply extends into movement, transforming maintenance into a continuous state of cultivation.

The term Qigong is a compound word. Qi, often translated as vital life-force energy, or simply breath. In Traditional Chinese Medicine, Qi is the invisible energy that animates the body, flows through the meridian system, and determines vitality. Your breath is viewed as the most direct way to cultivate and manage this vital Qi. Gong means skill, cultivation, or work. Therefore, Qigong literally means working with the breath-energy or the cultivation of life-force skill. It is the realisation that health is not something you acquire but something you work at, using the simplest tool you have: the breath.

The core idea of Qigong is to dissolve the division between practice and life. It is the art of performing every task, motion, and moment with a calm, deliberate, and nasal breath. Instead of performing exercises for a fixed 10 minutes, the Qigong mindset encourages you to do everything with a calm, nasal breath. The moment your breath becomes shallow, fast, or shifts to the mouth, your body is signalling a shift into the stress-dominant sympathetic state. By returning to slow, nasal breathing while you work, drive, or sit, you consciously keep the nervous system anchored in the restorative parasympathetic state.

All Qigong movements are performed in synchronisation with the breath. The motion is never forced or rushed; it flows from the inhale and exhale. This integration creates a moving meditation, reinforcing the parasympathetic signal and ensuring that physical work is restorative rather than depleting. When movements are executed slowly and smoothly, coordinated with the breath, they apply gentle, prolonged tensile stress to the fascial network. This deliberate, unhurried movement encourages fascial hydration, reduces internal friction, and enhances the flow of Qi and blood throughout the connective tissues.

A crucial, often-overlooked component of functional breathing is the proper tongue position. The correct, resting tongue posture places the tip gently against the hard palate, right behind the front teeth, with the body of the tongue pressed softly up against the entire roof of the mouth. This position seals the oral cavity, automatically preventing mouth-breathing. It activates the vagal circuit by engaging muscles and fascial pathways in the back of the throat and neck. And in the energetic framework of Qigong, it is said to complete the electrical circuit between the Governing Meridian running up the spine and the Conception Meridian running down the front of the body, allowing Qi to circulate smoothly.

You do not need to master complex postures to practise Qigong. You only need to adopt the mindset: your breath is your life-force, and the quality of your life is the direct result of the quality of your breath-work. Should you wish to pursue specific forms, there are countless resources, teachers, and online modules available.

The Liquid Matrix

Hydration and Nutritional Support for Fascia

Your fascial health is governed by three fundamental pillars: mechanical movement, neurological balance, and chemical support. While fascia-puncture and movement address the first two, the health of the entire system fundamentally relies on the third. The body's connective tissue is not a dry, static web; it is a dynamic, fluid matrix.

The true magic of fascia lies in its Extracellular Matrix, the non-cellular substance in which collagen and elastin fibres are embedded. The ECM, often called the ground substance, is primarily composed of water – fascia can store up to 23 percent of the body's total water – and a gel-like mixture of molecules. The key components are the Glycosaminoglycans and Proteoglycans, most notably Hyaluronan. These molecules are fiercely hydrophilic –

they love water – and their job is to bind massive amounts of water, creating a viscous, slippery gel.

When healthy and hydrated, this ground substance acts as a lubricant and a cushion. It allows the individual fascial layers, muscles, and organs to glide and slide over one another without friction. This fluidity is essential for effortless movement and the transmission of force. When unhealthy and dehydrated, the ground substance loses its water content, becoming thick, dense, and sticky. This dryness causes the delicate collagen fibres to clump together and form aberrant cross-links. This is the physical manifestation of restriction – the stiffness and discomfort that you feel.

For fascia to remain supple and responsive, it requires a steady, consistent supply of water. Sip, do not chug – your fascia needs a steady trickle throughout the day, rather than large, infrequent surges. Water-rich foods – cucumbers, celery, melon, and citrus fruits – provide water bound with electrolytes and nutrients, which is arguably more bioavailable to your tissues than plain tap water. And most importantly: movement is the hydration pump. Water alone is not enough; you must move to hydrate your fascia. The mechanical pressure from movement, stretching, and fascia-puncture techniques physically pumps the ground substance, forcing water into and out of the tissue layers. This process is essential for flushing metabolic waste and drawing fresh, clean fluid into the matrix.

To truly transform your health from within, you must treat your body's liquid matrix with as much care as your physical structure. The simple, daily choice of what you drink and what you eat is the chemical Qigong that ensures your fascia remains a flowing, adaptable, and healthy web.

Fluid Movement

Self-Care Techniques for Fascial Release

The work of fascia-puncture – or any deep bodywork – is only the first step. The true transformation happens in the space between treatments. If you return to old movement patterns and neglect your body, the restrictions will return. This chapter provides a toolkit of active self-care techniques designed to mobilise the fascial web, distribute hydration, and reinforce the neurological calm achieved through breathwork. These practices are not strenuous exercises; they are forms of Fluid Movement that use the principles of long-hold tension and gentle, rhythmic motion to keep your fascia supple and responsive.

Most people stretch muscles, which involves brief, intense pulls of 10 to 30 seconds, leading to a sharp pull at the end-range barrier. To truly influence the fascia, you must change your approach: the key to fascial release is applying a low and gentle load held for a significantly longer duration — a minimum of 90 to 120 seconds. The resulting sensation should not be a sharp pull, but rather a dull ache, a feeling of melting, or spreading warmth, which indicates you are engaging the connective tissue rather than just the muscle belly.

The Fascial Melt Technique: Find the barrier – move into a comfortable stretch. Stop at the first sense of tension, well before discomfort. Breathe into the stretch by adopting the LSD nasal breathing rhythm. Hold and wait for a minimum of 90 seconds. The extended time allows the viscous ground substance to begin to soften and release its adhesive cross-links. You will notice the tension gradually recede, allowing you to move slightly deeper without forcing. Exit slowly – the transition out is as important as the stretch itself.

Self-Myofascial Release uses tools like foam rollers, massage balls, and lacrosse balls to apply sustained pressure to specific fascial trigger points – areas of localised tension where your fascia has become dense, stuck, and potentially painful. Focus on common tension areas: the gluteal muscles, the outer thigh and IT band, the upper back and shoulder blades, and the soles of the feet. Apply low-to-moderate pressure. Anchor on the point of tension and hold for 30 to 60 seconds while using slow, nasal breathing. This sustained mechanical pressure forces fluids back into the localised area, helping the ECM to rehydrate.

Heat application is the most direct way to support the fluidity of the fascial system externally. The ground substance is a colloidal gel, meaning its viscosity is highly sensitive to temperature. Applying heat – through a hot bath, a heating pad, or a sauna – increases the kinetic energy of the molecules, making the gel instantly more fluid, much like how honey thins when warmed. This reduction in viscosity enhances tissue glide, promotes local circulation, aids waste removal, and prepares the tissue for deeper, more effective stretching and movement.

PART TWO

The Fascial Mind

Where Neuroscience Ends and Wisdom Begins
— Steve Brandl

How sensation, prediction, emotion, and the self-model meet the physical body. The Investigation is adapted from The Uncarved Block: An Encounter with Laozi & Zhuangzi; the chapters that follow draw on The Storytelling Monkey and the Web of Life.

The Investigation

What you are before the story begins

1 — *The Problem with Maps*

You are holding a map. You have been holding one since before you could speak. Not a paper map — something more intimate, more pervasive, and considerably more difficult to put down. A model of the world assembled by your nervous system from the first moments of extrauterine life, continuously revised, relentlessly maintained, and so thoroughly integrated into your experience that you mistake it, at every moment, for the territory itself. This is not a metaphor. The neuroscience is specific. Your brain does not passively receive reality and report it to you. It generates a model — a prediction of what is most likely to be happening — and serves that prediction up as your experience. What you see, hear, feel, and believe yourself to be is not the raw data. It is the brain's best guess, presented with such seamless authority that questioning it requires a deliberate act of investigation most people never perform. The philosopher Alfred Korzybski said it in 1931: the map is not the territory. He was more right than he knew. The map is so good, so continuously updated, so indistinguishable from what it represents, that we do not experience ourselves as holding a map at all. We experience ourselves as standing in the territory. We experience ourselves as the territory. This is the first thing the Daodejing asks you to see. Not as a philosophical position to be debated, but as something you can verify in your own experience, right now, in this moment.

What a Name Does

When you name something, you have done something more consequential than you realise. You have drawn a line around a portion of experience, separated it from everything else, and filed it under a category your nervous system already possesses. The thing named is no longer encountered freshly. It is recognised – which means, literally, cognised again, processed through existing templates, stripped of whatever does not fit the category, and delivered to your awareness as a known quantity. A tree. You read the word and something happened. Not a sensory encounter with a living organism – its particular bark, its specific weight of light through its specific leaves, the way it holds the ground in this specific wind – but a category activation. The label arrived before the perception could. This is how naming works. It is efficient, essential for survival, and it costs you almost everything. The Daodejing opens with this observation. The name that can be named is not the lasting name. It is a precise description of what happens when the map claims to be the territory. The named world is a managed world. A pre-digested world. A world in which the brain's filing system has already decided what everything is before you have a chance to encounter it directly.

There is a different kind of knowing. Not the absence of naming – we are linguistic creatures and the maps are not going away – but the recognition that the map is a map. The moment you see the label as a label, something shifts. Not dramatically. Quietly. The grip loosens by exactly one degree. And in that single degree of loosening, something becomes available that was not available a moment before: the thing itself, prior to what you called it.

The Monkey

Throughout this book I use a term that needs introducing before we go further: the Monkey. It is not a metaphor for something vague. It is a name for something specific –

the neural narrative apparatus that generates, without your permission and before your conscious awareness, a plausible account of who you are, what the world contains, and what you should do next. The neuroscientist Michael Gazzaniga, working with split-brain patients, discovered a module in the left hemisphere he called the Interpreter: a system whose sole function is to construct a coherent story about why the organism just did what it did – even when the actual cause is entirely hidden from it. The Interpreter does not deliberate. It confabulates, with complete conviction and zero awareness that the story is invented. The decision is made, the action is taken, the emotion arises – and then the Interpreter drafts the account. The account always arrives after the fact. But from the inside, it feels as if it arrived first.

This is the Monkey. Not a metaphor for irrationality. Not the opposite of reason. The biological inheritance that runs on neural hardware largely unchanged since the emergence of behaviourally modern humans – perhaps sixty to a hundred thousand years ago – now navigating a world of performance reviews, social media, and the peculiar modern suffering of knowing too much and feeling too little. You are not a rational being who occasionally lets emotion cloud judgement. You are a storytelling organism who, on occasion, achieves rationality. The story is always first. The Monkey builds your world before you can think. It claims authorship of decisions already made. It constructs the experience of you from moment to moment with the seamless confidence of a system that has never been asked to doubt itself. Seeing it clearly – not to silence it, but to recognise its narration as narration rather than truth – is the precondition for everything the Daodejing has to offer. Every chapter that follows, in both the investigation and the ancient text, is another angle on this question: what becomes possible when the Monkey's stories become something you carry, rather than something that carries you?

The Cost of Certainty

Here is what the investigation has taught me, after twenty years of working with the body and several years of sitting with this text: certainty is expensive. Not wrong — expensive. Every conviction you hold is a prediction your nervous system has committed to, and every committed prediction narrows the range of what you are capable of perceiving. The more certain you are, the less you see. This is not a character flaw. It is the operating principle of the predictive brain. Karl Friston's Free Energy Principle formalises this: the brain minimises surprise by maintaining the models it has learned to trust, even when those models are the source of the suffering. A patient who has carried the story of their body as fragile for twenty years does not perceive the same shoulder that an MRI reveals. They perceive the shoulder their model predicts — guarded, restricted, one wrong movement from catastrophe. The tissue may have healed years ago. The model has not. The Daodejing offers the same observation without the mathematics. The sage diminishes daily. What is diminished, in Friston's terms, are the priors – the accumulated certainties that have thickened into walls. What remains when the walls thin is not nothing. It is the opposite of nothing. It is the capacity to encounter what is actually here, before the model has told you what it should be. I have watched this happen in the treatment room. A tissue releases that has been held for years, and the patient goes quiet – not the quiet of relaxation, but the quiet of something unfamiliar arriving. The model expected tension. The absence of tension is, for a moment, genuinely new. In that moment, before the Monkey narrates it into a category, the patient is closer to what the Daodejing points at than any amount of reading could have brought them. Then the narration arrives, and the moment is filed. But the body remembers. The body always remembers.

2 – *The Self You Think You Are*

If the map is not the territory, then the most intimate map of all – the one you call yourself — deserves the closest examination. This is where the investigation becomes uncomfortable, and where most people decide to return to the safety of their existing beliefs. I am asking you not to do that. Not because discomfort is virtuous, but because what lies on the other side of this particular discomfort is worth the crossing. You carry, at every moment, a felt sense of being someone. A continuous, coherent I that wakes up in the morning, moves through the day, and falls asleep at night, fundamentally the same person it was yesterday. This sense is so intimate, so uninterrupted, so absolutely convincing from the inside, that questioning it feels not merely counterintuitive but almost dangerous — as though pulling on this thread might unravel something essential. The neuroscience suggests otherwise. What the brain produces is not a self but a self-model — a continuously updated representation that Thomas Metzinger calls the phenomenal self. It is a process, not a thing. An ongoing construction, not a discovered entity. And its most remarkable property is what Metzinger calls transparency: the model does not present itself as a model. There is no watermark. No border. No moment where the brain says: this is my best current guess about who you are. It simply delivers the experience of being someone, seamlessly, and you take it – as you have always taken it – for the unmediated truth.

What Laozi Saw Without the Scanner

Twenty-five centuries before neuroimaging, Laozi described this with a precision that still startles me. The sage has no fixed self, he wrote. He takes the hearts of the people as his own heart. This is not altruism. It is a description of what the self actually is when you stop insisting it is something solid. The sage is not selfless in the moral sense of sacrificing personal desire for others. The sage is selfless in the structural sense of having seen through the model – having recognised the I as a construction, useful but not ultimate, and therefore no longer imprisoned by its demands. This is not an easy thing to understand, and it is an even harder thing to experience. The Monkey – the neural narrative apparatus – has been constructing this self since before you could speak. Every memory, every preference, every fear and aspiration has been woven into a story so compelling that separating yourself from it feels like dying. In a sense, it is. Not the death of the organism, but the death of a conviction – the conviction that the story and the storyteller are the same thing. The Daodejing returns to this, again and again, with different images. Water, which has no fixed shape and takes the form of whatever contains it. The valley, which receives everything precisely because it is empty. The uncarved block, which can become anything because it has not yet been made into something specific. These are not metaphors for a philosophical position. They are descriptions of what it is like, from the inside, when the self-model loosens its grip.

The Freedom in Not Knowing

There is a particular quality of not-knowing that the Western intellectual tradition handles badly. We are trained to treat uncertainty as a problem — a temporary state to be resolved by better information, sharper analysis, more rigorous method. And for many questions, this is exactly right. You want your surgeon to be certain about which side to operate on. You want your engineer to be certain about the load-bearing capacity of the bridge. But there is another kind of not-knowing — the kind that arrives when you have followed an honest investigation as far as it goes and discovered that the question itself is larger than any answer you can construct. This is not ignorance. It is not intellectual laziness. It is the specific epistemic humility that comes from having done the work and found the edge. The Daodejing begins here. Its first line is not a statement of doctrine but a warning: the way that can be spoken is not the lasting way. Laozi is not being coy. He is being precise. What he is pointing at cannot be captured in a proposition, because every proposition is a map, and what he is pointing at is the territory prior to all maps. Not the territory as opposed to the map — that would just be another map, labelled the real thing. The territory as it is before the labelling begins. Before the story starts. Before you arrive with your filing system and your categories and your urgent need to know what this is. I have spent most of my intellectual life building maps. Good maps, I believe. Maps that have helped patients, that have organised genuine insight, that have brought the neuroscience and the ancient wisdom into productive contact. But the deepest thing the Daodejing has taught me is not on any of those maps. It is the quiet that arrives when I put the maps down. Not the quiet of emptiness – the quiet of fullness so complete that no description is adequate. The Daodejing has a word for it. It calls it the mystery. I have learned not to try to name it further than that.

3 – *Opposites and the Trap Between Them*

The mind divides. This is what it does. Before you have taken your first conscious step into the day, the brain has already sorted the incoming data into categories: safe and unsafe, pleasant and unpleasant, self and not-self, known and unknown. This sorting is so fast, so automatic, so deeply embedded in the neural architecture, that by the time you are aware of experiencing anything, the division has already occurred. You do not experience the world and then judge it. You experience a world that has already been judged. The Daodejing's second chapter makes this its subject. When everyone knows beauty as beauty, ugliness has already been born. When everyone knows good as good, not-good has already awakened. This is not a moral observation. It is a structural one. The moment you draw a line, you create two sides. The moment you name one side, you have implicitly defined the other. Every act of distinction is simultaneously an act of division. This would be merely interesting as philosophy if it did not have such specific consequences in how we live. But it does. The person who pursues happiness with great determination creates, with that very determination, a precise and detailed map of unhappiness — everything that happiness is not, everything that stands between them and the goal, every way the current moment fails to match the desired one. The pursuit does not move them toward happiness. It moves them deeper into the structure of opposition itself, where happiness and unhappiness define each other endlessly and neither can exist without the other.

The Third Position

What the Daodejing points toward is not a resolution of opposites but something harder and more interesting: a position that is not a position. Not choosing one side over the other. Not balancing between them. Not even synthesising them into some higher unity. Something prior to the division itself – the ground from which the distinction arose, and which was never divided. In clinical practice, I encounter this constantly. A patient arrives with pain on one side and tension on the other, and the temptation – both theirs and mine – is to fix the problem, which means to eliminate the pain and preserve the comfort. But the pain and the tension are not separate problems. They are two expressions of a single pattern – a holding pattern the nervous system adopted, years ago, for reasons that made perfect sense at the time. To release one side without addressing the pattern is to create a new imbalance. To address the pattern is to work with the whole system, prior to the division into pain-here and compensation-there. This is what Laozi means by Wu Wei — a term mistranslated as inaction so frequently that its actual meaning has been almost completely obscured. Wu Wei is not passivity. It is action that does not fight the pattern. Action that does not begin from a position of opposition to what is. Action that arises from the same ground the problem arose from, and therefore has access to the whole system rather than one warring half of it. The sage acts without contending. Not because contention is morally wrong, but because contention can only reach one side of a divide it has already accepted. The sage reaches both sides by not starting from either one.

4 — *What the Body Knows*

Twenty years of clinical practice have taught me something that no amount of reading could have: the body holds what the mind has not yet named. This is not a poetic claim. It is a clinical observation, made thousands of times, in the tissue of patients who carry in their fascia the precise contour of experiences their conscious narrative has never included. A woman comes in with chronic tension in her right shoulder. The tension is specific — a particular quality of holding, a particular depth, a particular relationship to the breath. As the tissue releases under sustained pressure, she begins to cry. Not from pain. From recognition. Something is surfacing that has been held, silently and faithfully, in the tissue for years. She does not need to name it for the release to occur. In fact, naming it too quickly — rushing to construct a narrative about what the crying means — can interrupt the process. The body is doing its own work. The mind's job, for once, is to stay out of the way. The Daodejing calls this the intelligence of the valley — the low place that receives everything without grasping, that holds without possessing, that allows without controlling. The body is this valley. It holds what the story-making mind has overlooked, suppressed, or simply not had the language for. And it holds it with a fidelity that the conscious narrative, with all its revisions and self-serving edits, cannot match.

The Fascial Web as Living Memory

The fascia – the continuous web of connective tissue that wraps every muscle, organ, nerve, and bone in the body – is not inert scaffolding. It is a sensory organ, dense with mechanoreceptors, capable of responding to mechanical force, emotional state, and sustained postural patterns by reorganising its molecular structure. What this means in practice is that the body does not merely hold postures. It becomes them. A shoulder held in guarded tension for five years is not simply a muscle that needs to relax. It is a fascial architecture that has been remodelled, at the molecular level, to support that pattern. This is why a single instruction to relax is almost never sufficient. The tissue has been restructured around the holding. The nervous system's predictive model expects the tension. Both the map and the territory have adapted to the pattern. To change the pattern requires working at both levels simultaneously – new input to the tissue and new prediction for the nervous system. The Daodejing understood this without the molecular biology. It speaks of returning to the root – not as a nostalgic retreat to some original state, but as a recognition that the deepest change comes not from adding something new but from releasing what was added unnecessarily. The uncarved block is not a blank slate. It is the living potential that was present before the carving began. The body knows this. The body has always known this. The mind is usually the last to arrive.

5 – *Standing at the Gate*

There is a place the investigation reaches where the tools that brought you here can take you no further. Not because the tools are inadequate – they have done extraordinary work, mapping the nervous system, tracing the predictive hierarchy, following the body's intelligence into the fascia and beyond. But because what lies beyond this point is not the kind of thing a tool can reach. A tool works by grasping. What lies beyond the gate does not submit to being grasped. The philosopher David Chalmers named this boundary the Hard Problem of Consciousness: the question of why physical processes give rise to subjective experience at all. You can describe every synapse, every neurotransmitter, every network activation with perfect precision, and you will still not have explained why any of it feels like something from the inside. The feeling – the warmth of it, the absolute immediacy, the irreducible first-person fact that there is something it is like to be you – remains outside the reach of the third-person description. Not temporarily. Structurally. This is where the investigation becomes genuinely interesting. Not because the gap is a problem to be solved, but because it is the most honest place in human thought. Every tradition of genuine inquiry has arrived here. The ones that pretend to have crossed it are selling something. The ones that stand in front of it honestly – the ones that acknowledge the limit without retreating from it – are the ones worth listening to.

The Daodejing is one of these. It arrived at this gate two millennia ago and, instead of constructing an elaborate theology to explain what lies beyond it, said simply: the mystery. Dark upon dark. The gate of all wonders. And then it turned around and offered eighty-one chapters of practical wisdom about how to live well on this side of the gate – in a world that is simultaneously mapped and unmappable, known and unknowable, named and forever beyond naming. This is the text that runs beneath everything in this book – including, in its own way, the practices that follow. Not because I have understood it – I have not, and anyone who claims to has not either. But because the encounter with it has changed how I see, how I practice, and how I hold the questions that the science alone could not resolve. The investigation does not end at the gate. It changes character. It becomes less about accumulation and more about release. Less about knowing and more about the quality of not-knowing that remains when the Monkey has exhausted its stories. That quality is what the Daodejing has been pointing at from its first word. And it is available, right now, in this moment, to anyone willing to stop pretending they already know what it is.

If the brain constructs a model of the self, then the next question for a fascia-puncturist is unavoidable: where does that model meet the physical body? Fascia.

The Feelings Within

Exploring the Emotional Link

Our bodies are so much more than just a collection of muscles, bones, and organs. They are vessels that carry not only our physical being but also our emotional selves. And these two aspects are deeply intertwined. When we experience emotions, they do not just stay in our minds; they often find their way into our physical bodies, becoming woven into the very fabric of our tissues. This is particularly true with fascia, that vast and interconnected web that permeates every part of us. In this chapter, we explore the profound connection between our emotions and our fascia, and how addressing that connection can be a powerful aspect of healing.

It is common to say things like "I am carrying the weight of the world on my shoulders" or "I feel tied up in knots." These are not just figures of speech; they often reflect a physical reality. When we experience stress, anxiety, grief, or unresolved anger, these emotions can translate into physical tension, especially in our muscles and fascia.

Think about it: when you are stressed, what happens to your body? Do your shoulders creep up towards your ears? Do you clench your jaw? Does your stomach feel tight? These are all examples of how our emotions can manifest physically. This is no mere temporary phenomenon. If we consistently hold these tensions, they can become ingrained in our tissues, creating chronic restrictions and affecting our posture, movement, and even our pain levels.

Fascia, with its extensive sensory network and its ability to respond to tension and stress, can become a sort of repository for our emotional holding patterns. When we suppress or ignore our feelings, that energy does not simply disappear; it can get stored in our tissues. The muscles might tense up, and the fascia surrounding those muscles can thicken and become restricted. These restrictions can limit movement, cause pain, and even affect the flow of blood and energy through the body.

The neuroscience behind this process is increasingly well understood. Antonio Damasio's somatic marker hypothesis demonstrated that the brain continuously reads the body's physiological state — patterns of tension, arousal, ease, and restriction registered in the muscles, viscera, and connective tissue — and uses these somatic markers as the primary basis for evaluating options and guiding choice. Emotion is not an interference with rational thought. It is the biological substrate in which rational thought is embedded. A chronic fascial restriction is therefore not merely a structural problem. It is a persistent somatic marker – a signal the brain continuously reads and incorporates into its model of who this person is and what their world permits.

Imagine a tightly woven fishing net. When the net is stretched and strained in certain areas, those areas become tighter and less flexible, while other parts might be left loose. Similarly, when we hold emotional tension in certain parts of our body, the corresponding areas of fascia become tighter and less pliable, affecting the overall integrity of the web.

This connection between emotions and fascia becomes particularly evident during treatments like fascia-puncture. As we release physical restrictions in the tissue, we sometimes also unlock emotional releases. A patient might suddenly feel a wave of sadness or grief, or they might start laughing uncontrollably. These are not random occurrences; they are often the emotional energy that has been held in the tissues being freed.

It is as if by addressing the physical tension, we are also opening a door to the emotions that have been locked away. This can be a powerful and transformative experience, allowing patients to process and release emotions they might not have even been consciously aware of. It is not about forcing emotions to the surface, but rather creating a safe space for them to emerge naturally as the body unwinds.

When these emotional releases happen, it is essential to approach them with compassion and respect. Simply holding space, listening, and offering a supportive presence can be incredibly helpful. For the practitioner, it is important to be aware of this possibility and to be prepared. It is not our role to be therapists or to analyse the patient's emotions, but rather to witness and support their experience. We trust that the body knows what it needs to release.

Ultimately, this exploration highlights the interconnectedness of our physical and emotional selves. We cannot truly address physical pain or dysfunction without also acknowledging the potential role of emotions. And similarly, working with the body can be a powerful way to access and release emotions held deep within.

This integration of the physical and emotional is key to holistic healing. It reminds us that fascia is more than just a physical structure; it is also a repository for our emotional experiences. By acknowledging and respecting this emotional link, we can create a more profound approach to healing through fascia-puncture and other bodywork modalities. We are not just treating the tissues; we are honouring the whole person — body, mind, and spirit.

The Breath-Body Link

Releasing Trapped Emotion and Fascial Tension

If the brain is the narrative engine of our lives, the fascia is the body's quiet, diligent recorder. It is a biological truth that intense, unresolved emotions — fear, grief, chronic anxiety, and trauma – do not simply vanish; they are logged as patterns of physical restriction within the body's connective tissue matrix.

When we face stress or emotional upheaval, the body's primal reaction is to mobilise for survival: muscles tense, the heart rate accelerates, and – crucially – the breathing becomes shallow, rapid, and often confined to the upper chest. This reflex is a neurological brace, designed to limit movement and conserve energy, which scientists call the freeze or tonic immobility response.

When this stress is chronic, this protective posture becomes permanent. The fascia, rich in nerve endings, tightens and shortens around these frozen patterns, becoming a silent reservoir for emotional energy. This chronic restriction creates adhesions, hindering movement, impacting structural integrity, and manifesting as pain, stiffness, or a general sense of being stuck.

The goal of true healing, therefore, is not just to release the physical restriction, but to create a pathway for the underlying emotional energy to move and be safely discharged.

Interoception and the Vagal Signal of Safety

To release emotions stored in the fascia, we must first learn to listen to the body. This is the domain of interoception: the conscious awareness of internal bodily states, such as heart rate, gut activity, and muscular tension.

The primary neural conduit for interoception is the Vagus Nerve. This nerve is a bidirectional highway, sending vast amounts of sensory information from the organs, fascia, and gut to the brain. It is the vagus nerve that informs the brain about the body's current state – safe and calm, or threatened and mobilised.

When chronic stress or trauma has dominated, the vagal tone is often low, and interoception is poor. The nervous system becomes dysregulated, losing its ability to accurately sense the internal environment and modulate emotions. This is where functional breathing becomes a powerful therapeutic tool.

The LSD Breath as the Fascial Solvent

Practising the same Light, Slow, Deep breathing described earlier in this book directly engages the vagus nerve and restores this regulatory capacity. In the specific context of trauma release, its three elements do something more precise than general relaxation: lightness signals safety to a hyper-vigilant system, slowness shifts the balance from sympathetic toward parasympathetic dominance, and depth gives the diaphragm's full three-dimensional movement room to mobilise the deep fascial connections — running from the lumbar spine, where fear and tension often anchor, up through the core canister — that a freeze response has locked in place.

During a fascia-puncture session, or even in a moment of emotional processing, a conscious switch to LSD breathing can initiate a Somatic Emotional Response. The act of breathing deep into a restricted area, previously held in a freeze response, helps the tissue and the trapped energy to unwind. The stored emotion is liberated – often as a spontaneous tear, tremor, or surge of heat – because the nervous system has finally been given the signal: it is safe to let go.

This intentional, compassionate use of breath transforms the physical release of fascia into a profound emotional and spiritual healing. It is the vital key to transforming health from within.

Beyond the Physical - When Emotions Speak Through Your Body

Despite remarkable advancements in physiotherapy and sports medicine, many individuals continue to experience persistent or recurring pain conditions that show only fleeting or minimal improvement with conventional treatments. In such cases, particularly when pain and discomfort arise without a clear physical injury or structural damage, it is crucial to consider a significant underlying factor: our emotions.

We all intuitively understand the powerful link between our feelings and our physical responses. Think of the clenched jaw during moments of intense stress, the balled fists or tightened shoulders that accompany anger. These are just surface-level examples of a deeper connection. When powerful emotions, especially anger and stress, are consistently suppressed, they do not simply vanish. Instead, they can become somatised, held within our tissues through the intricate workings of our subconscious mind. Like a skilled projector, the unconscious mind can divert our attention from these unresolved negative emotions by manifesting them as physical symptoms: muscle contractions, fascial tension, and even the constriction of blood vessels. These physiological changes, though often perceived as alarming, are fundamentally harmless attempts by the body to distract from the emotional burden. They can lead to increased pressure on sensitive nerve endings and a subtle reduction in oxygen supply to the soft tissues. I call these unconscious processes Emotional Myofascial Tensions – EMFT.

Since writing the first edition of this book, I have had the opportunity to explore the neuroscience behind EMFT more deeply, particularly through the research that also became the foundation of Part II of this book. The framework I call EMFT is my own synthesis, developed across twenty years of clinical observation, though the underlying insights build on established work: Wilhelm Reich's concept of character armour, Peter Levine's somatic experiencing approach, Bessel van der Kolk's research on how trauma is stored in the body, and Antonio Damasio's somatic marker hypothesis. What the fascial framework adds is clinical specificity – a way of locating where in the connective matrix a given emotional pattern has taken up residence, and what the tissue responds to when that pattern is addressed directly.

The brain, as Anil Seth has demonstrated, is fundamentally a prediction machine. It does not passively receive sensory information; it generates its best model of what is most likely happening and compares that model against incoming data. Karl Friston's Free Energy Principle proposes that the fundamental drive of any living system is to minimise surprise – to maintain its existing model. The brain's Default Mode Network – the neural substrate of self-referential thought – is where this model lives. When the DMN runs without interruption, the narrative becomes rigid. Past failures arrive as current evidence. Future threats present themselves as certainties. And the fascia, rich in sensory receptors feeding into this predictive system, becomes both the evidence for the story and the medium in which the story is physically maintained. Part II of this book returns to this mechanism – the Monkey's predictive architecture – in far greater depth.

When anger is not expressed – when it becomes a background condition rather than an acute response – the muscles of the shoulder girdle, neck, and jaw do not simply return to neutral. They contract, repeatedly, and the fascia adapts to that sustained contraction: thickening, shortening, settling into the architecture of the held state. The emotional pattern has been written into tissue. The anger is no longer only a psychological event. It has become a posture, a restriction, a characteristic configuration of the liquid connective matrix. Grief takes up residence differently — in the anterior chain, in the rounding of the shoulders, in the shortened pectoral fascia that pulls the body into the posture of collapse. Fear settles into the diaphragm and the psoas, bracing the body against a threat that may have passed years ago.

Drawing from my own experiences navigating the joys and challenges of early fatherhood, I can offer a relatable example. The demands of caring for a newborn, coupled with a partner equally navigating the stresses of new parenthood, can sometimes lead to feelings of being overlooked or unheard. The baby's persistent crying can amplify feelings of helplessness and frustration. Anger may arise, yet expressing it towards a vulnerable infant or an already overwhelmed partner is often unthinkable. This unexpressed anger, swallowed repeatedly, can then be projected by the unconscious mind, manifesting as unexplained aches and pains in the body. Similarly, unresolved conflicts with a boss, partner, parents, or other significant individuals can lead to the chronic storage of anger and resentment within the body's tissues. Common areas for these emotional projections include the back, neck, shoulders, and hips. However, EMFT can also manifest as numbness in the arms or legs, or gastrointestinal disturbances like acid reflux or indigestion.

If you suspect that EMFT might be contributing to, or even the root cause of, your pain or discomfort, there is an accessible first step: acceptance. Consider incorporating the following mantra into your daily routine, repeating it several times a day or whenever your symptoms are most prominent:

"I accept that my pain is caused, or increased, by repressed emotions. My subconscious mind is projecting stored unresolved emotions into Myofascial Tensions and blood vessel contractions, causing mild oxygen deprivation and pressure on free nerve endings. This is a harmless condition, and I have nothing to fear. By accepting my emotions as the root of my pain, I take control over my unconscious mind and stop this projection."

Furthermore, consciously remind yourself whenever negative emotions arise: "I will not allow my subconscious mind to project this emotion into physical pain."

A shorter version: "I accept my emotions as the root of my pain. I take control over my unconscious mind and stop this projection of Myofascial tensions."

You have little to lose by consistently applying this technique for one to three months. Many individuals report noticeable shifts in their pain perception within days to weeks. Besides the power of acceptance, keeping an emotional journal to track feelings and identify patterns can bring valuable awareness. Creating a list of both present and past negative emotions, though it may become extensive, is also helpful.

On a lighter note, some find it helpful to engage directly with their subconscious mind, even having a conversation or playfully yelling at it to cease the painful projections. Try speaking to your reflection in the mirror each morning. In cases involving severe trauma or deeply rooted emotional issues, seeking professional support through psychotherapy is a necessary and transformative step.

Clinical Insights

Applying Fascia-Puncture – Illustrative Patient Journeys

Mr. A's migraines opened this book, in the chapter that introduced this practice. The cases that follow – Ms. B's foot pain, Mr. C's acute elbow injury, Ms. D's journey through miscarriage to pregnancy, and Ms. E's transformative experience with chronic pain – extend the same principles across a wider range of presentations. This method is characterised by a holistic and meticulous assessment, integrating comprehensive patient history, refined palpation skills, and a deep understanding of fascial interconnectedness. It champions precision in needling, not merely in location but also in angle and depth, always adaptable to the unique needs of the tissue and the patient's evolving response. Furthermore, it explicitly acknowledges and integrates the interplay of physical and emotional states, fostering an environment where deep-seated tensions, both somatic and psychological, can be safely released. Ultimately, fascia-puncture is presented not just as a technique for pain relief, but as a systematic methodology designed to restore the body's inherent balance, resilience, and vitality, unlocking new levels of well-being from within.

Ms. B presented with a chief complaint of severe pain in her left foot, meticulously localised to the region between the third and fourth interdigital nerves. This pain, rated at an excruciating 7 to 8 out of 10, was consistently exacerbated immediately upon waking and after prolonged standing or walking. She had been diagnosed with Morton's neuroma. Her presentation also included muscle soreness in the anterior and lateral ankle region attributed to compensatory pain avoidance behaviours.

Our treatment protocol began with two fascia-puncture sessions per week. After just three to four treatments, Ms. B reported a substantial reduction in foot pain, with the majority of her initial discomfort relieved. What remained was primarily a subtle morning achiness in the lateral ankle, which consistently subsided within a few minutes of light activity. This residual symptom illustrates the sponginess and dynamic nature of fascia. During inactivity, fascial tissues tend to accumulate metabolic waste and receive fewer fresh nutrients. Brief movement swiftly restores optimal blood flow, elasticity, and fluidity.

About 20 to 25 small Korean hand acupuncture needles were inserted directly into the affected interdigital spaces on both plantar and dorsal aspects. A few were also placed in adjacent interdigital spaces.

Standard needles were utilised on the anterior and lateral ankle regions, extending up the lower leg along the fascial connections, adding another 15 to 20 needles. After 15 total sessions with varying frequencies, the residual soreness had diminished to near zero.

Mr. C arrived with an acute onset of severe pain in his right elbow and wrist following a 90-minute badminton session. His medical history included a resolved episode of neck and shoulder pain two years prior and occasional low back fatigue from prolonged sitting.

Treatment began with three intensive fascia-puncture sessions over two weeks. Approximately 25 needles were placed within the arm during each session, along the lateral, posterior, and medial arm lines. An additional 15 needles addressed connections to both sides of the lateral neck and the right deltoid region. Furthermore, 15 to 20 more needles were strategically inserted into the lateral low back, pelvic, and hip regions on both sides, and the right

IT-band, peroneus, and lateral ankle were also treated. Each session involved 50 to 60 needles.

Following two weeks and a temporary break from badminton, Mr. C's elbow pain significantly subsided. He reported complete absence of low back fatigue and marked improvement in stress resistance. He resumed badminton without recurrence of acute pain. Maintenance sessions continued at decreasing frequency.

Ms. D sought assistance for a very personal concern. Three months prior, she had experienced a miscarriage during her third month of pregnancy. Her emotional resilience was remarkable, supported by engagement with support groups and her robust understanding, facilitated by her gynaecologist and husband, that miscarriages are a common experience. Her primary goals were to re-establish a balanced menstrual cycle and improve fertility. Prior to the miscarriage, her cycle typically spanned 27 to 29 days; it had recently become longer, significantly more painful, with heavier bleeding and increased moodiness. She also reported persistent tension in her neck and right shoulder.

Our healthcare plan was structured with 20 sessions across three menstrual cycles. The majority were conducted in a supine position, focusing on the lower abdominal and pelvic fascia with approximately 20 to 25 needles. Concurrently, 10 to 15 needles were placed on the medial aspects of the legs, addressing their direct fascial continuity through the internal pelvis and lower abdomen. Another 15 to 20 needles were applied to her neck and right shoulder.

Within three months, Ms. D's menstrual cycle had regained its normal rhythm. A further three months later, she joyfully conceived. This profoundly positive outcome highlights the power of addressing fascial connections related to internal organs and glands. I highly recommend resources like Luigi and Antonio Stecco's Fascial Manipulation for Internal Dysfunctions for practitioners seeking to deepen this area of expertise.

Ms. E visited primarily for protracted and debilitating heel pain, which had significantly impaired her daily activities for many months. She candidly acknowledged a history of neglecting her health in pursuit of career advancement. X-rays revealed heel spurs and calcific tendonitis of the Achilles tendons, more pronounced on the left side. She also experienced meralgia in her left leg. To mitigate work-related stress, treatment strategically included the fascia layers of the shoulders, neck, and head.

Our treatment protocol began with three fascia-puncture sessions per week for three weeks, followed by two sessions per week for another three weeks, then transitioning to longer-term maintenance. Sessions frequently involved 70 to 100 needles. Restrictions were treated across the anterior hip, lateral and anterior left leg, medial knee, and calf, with particular attention to the Achilles tendons. About 10 needles addressed abdominal fascia for digestion and weight management. Another 10 to 20 were placed in the trapezius, lateral occipital, anterior neck, and head fascia for stress-related tension.

During neck and head sessions, Ms. E often experienced profound emotional releases, manifesting as tears. She began to anticipate these releases, recognising their role in fostering greater balance. After just two to three weeks, she reported feeling like a new person: mobility dramatically improved, pain significantly subsided, and her motivation to manage her health became positive. She firmly established healthier exercise and nutritional routines. Ms. E embraced fascia-puncture as an integral part of her wellness routine, continuing to visit monthly. Alongside fascia-puncture, she received adjunctive therapies including massages and shockwave therapy.

A note on methodology: as an attentive reader may observe, I primarily conduct treatments in a single position at any given appointment – typically supine or prone, with occasional side-lying or sitting. I deliberately avoid switching positions and performing a second concurrent session, as I believe using numerous needles and shifting positions can potentially overwhelm a patient's inherent healing capacities.

A typical fascia-puncture session is structured to maximise benefit and comfort. An initial consultation lasts between 40 to 60 minutes: 10 to 15 minutes for examination, 10 to 15 for needle insertions, 15 to 20 for rest with needles in place, and 5 to 10 for removal. Subsequent sessions are more concise at 35 to 45 minutes.

These cases collectively underscore the fundamental principles: holistic assessment integrating comprehensive patient history, refined palpation, and deep understanding of fascial interconnectedness; precision in needling; integration of physical and emotional states; and systematic methodology designed to restore the body's inherent balance and vitality.

The Biotensegrity Model

Unifying Posture, Pain, and Puncture

We have already established that fascia forms a single continuous web. Biotensegrity is the model that explains what that continuity actually does mechanically – how a treatment applied to one part of your body can alleviate pain in a seemingly unrelated area. It requires moving beyond the conventional model of human mechanics, which views the body as a stack of compression-based parts: bones stacked on bones, muscles pulling levers, joints as simple hinges.

The modern, holistic view is the Biotensegrity Model. This concept provides the essential, unified understanding of posture, movement, and the global function of the fascial system, explaining the profound effectiveness of the fascia-puncture approach.

Biotensegrity is the application of the engineering principle of Tensegrity – Tensional Integrity – to biological structures. It is a system that balances continuous tension with discontinuous compression.

Continuous Tension is the role of the fascia – the entire connective tissue network – and all soft tissues. It forms a single, continuous, pre-stressed, elastic web, running from the deepest ligament to the most superficial layer of skin. This web keeps everything taut and integrated.

Discontinuous Compression is the role of the bones. They float in the tensional matrix, held apart by the pull of the surrounding soft tissue, and they never directly touch one another, except at joints, which are lubricated surfaces of movement.

The key insight: in a tensegrity structure, the structure is strengthened by its uniform distribution of force. When you apply pressure to one point, the entire network – not just the local area – must adjust to absorb and redistribute that force. The body is an integrated elastic shell, not a rigid, segmented machine.

In the Biotensegrity model, posture is not about standing up straight. Posture is the equilibrium of the continuous tensional web. A chronic restriction, perhaps from an old ankle sprain, a sedentary lifestyle, or emotional holding patterns, acts like a permanent shortening of a single rope within the global fascial net. This local tightness forces the entire network to compensate. The pull from the ankle might cause a tilt in the pelvis, which then forces the spine to curve to keep the head level, ultimately manifesting as chronic tension in the neck or jaw.

The site of pain is rarely the source of the problem. It is often the victim – the area where the fascial network has become excessively strained due to compensating for tightness elsewhere. The chronic lower back pain you feel might be a result of chronic tension in your Deep Front Line fascia, which begins in your feet.

The Biotensegrity framework explains why fascia-puncture is so effective and transformative. You are not treating the pain

– you are correcting the tension imbalance that caused the pain. The needle is used to locate and release a point of high, localised tension – an anchor point holding the global system out of balance. When the needle is manipulated at that specific fascial restriction, it causes a localised mechanical release – a softening of the ground substance and a micro-release of contracted cells. Because the fascia is a single, continuous web, this is my working model for what happens next: the localised release changes the tension picture the rest of the network is adjusting around, and – in my clinical experience – the wider system often re-equilibrates in response. This allows the floating compression elements – the bones – to settle into a more natural, low-strain position. The patient experiences this as an instantaneous release of tension in a distant area, greater range of motion, and a return to a more efficient, less painful postural state.

Ultimately, by treating the fascial net, you are speaking the language of Biotensegrity, shifting the body's entire tensional architecture toward a balanced, fluid, and self-supporting state.

PART THREE

The Practice

Fascia-puncture, breathing, palpation, self-work, and the practical integration of everything learned

Fascia-Puncture

Releasing the Body's Potential

Fascia-puncture is a specialised needling approach centred on addressing the pathophysiological changes within the fascial network to promote healing and restore optimal function. This technique involves the strategic placement of fine needles into specific points along myofascial meridians, guided by careful palpation to locate areas where restrictions or altered gliding ability are present. Through this targeted needle insertion, fascia-puncture aims to elicit several therapeutic effects that influence both the local tissue and the broader interconnected fascial system.

A key aspect of fascia-puncture lies in its capacity to provide mechanical stimulation and induce tissue relaxation. The insertion and gentle manipulation of needles can mechanically interact with the fascia, aiding in the breakdown of excessive collagen cross-links that contribute to stiffness, releasing restrictive adhesions between fascial layers, and ultimately improving the overall mobility and glide of the fascial network. The intended effect could be visualised as winding-up and lengthening collagen fibres to release tension, similar to how spaghetti is manipulated around a fork.

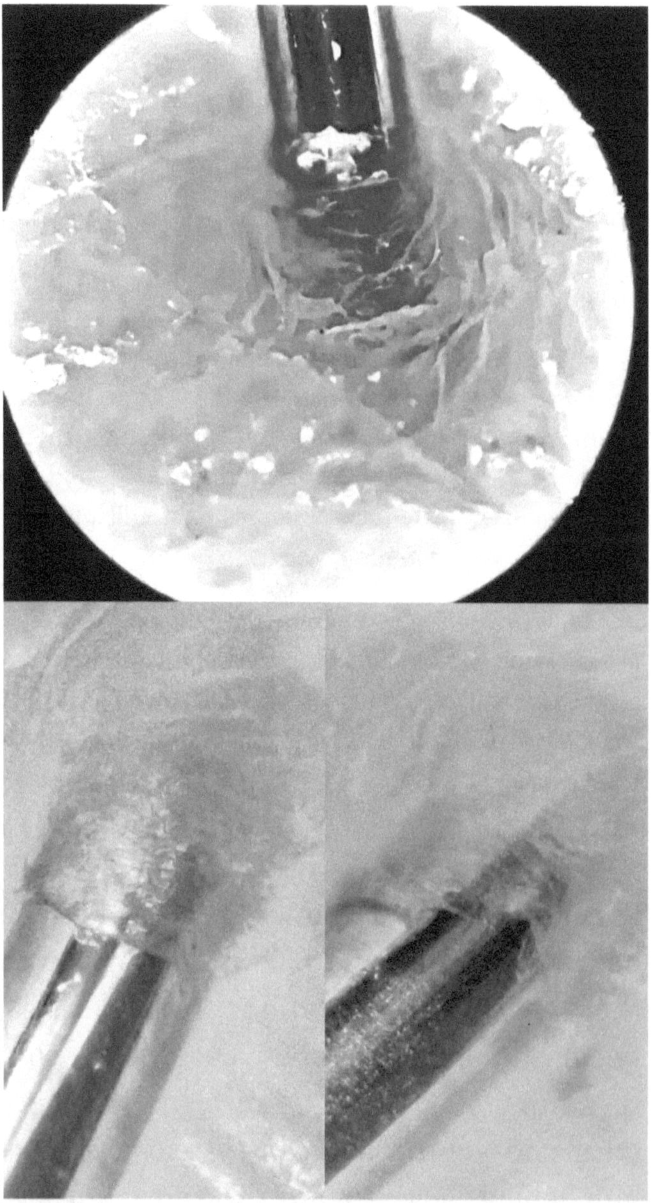

Figure 1: Fascial response to needle rotation observed with a handheld microscope. Images captured with a Carson MicroMini MM-300 Pocket Microscope attached to a Samsung Galaxy S23 FE smartphone. The acupuncture needle was inserted at the author's wrist near the point LI5 (Yangxi).

The micrographs illustrate the local fascial environment surrounding the needle tip. Collagen fibers and connective tissue structures appear to wind and gather around the needle shaft during manipulation. This phenomenon corresponds to the mechanical interaction between the needle and the fascial matrix, sometimes described as needle grasp or connective tissue winding.

Images were taken in vivo on the author's own body using a stabilized handheld microscope placed directly on the skin surface. The photographs were converted to black and white to enhance structural contrast for print reproduction.

Furthermore, fascia-puncture plays a role in neuromodulation and pain reduction. Given the rich innervation of fascia, needlestimulation directly engages sensory receptors, modulating pain signals at both local and central nervous system levels. By influencing nerve endings within the fascia, this technique can reduce pain perception and alleviate discomfort. The occasional electric twitch observed during treatment likely reflects a direct effect on local muscle and fascia, resulting in immediate relaxation and reduced pressure on pain-sensitive structures.

Improved blood flow and hydration are also significant outcomes. The needling action stimulates local circulation in the treated areas, delivering essential nutrients and oxygen to the tissues while simultaneously facilitating the removal of metabolic waste products and inflammatory mediators. This enhanced blood flow contributes to the rehydration of the ground substance, the gel-like matrix that lubricates fascial layers, which is crucial for restoring optimal fascial gliding.

Fascia-puncture also triggers the body's inherent healing mechanisms. The microtrauma caused by needle insertion initiates a localised healing response, prompting the release of growth factors and other signalling molecules that support tissue repair and regeneration within the fascia.

Beyond the physical effects, the release of fascial restrictions by fascia-puncture can have an emotional component. Patients may experience emotional releases, accompanied by feelings of lightness and clarity, highlighting the interconnectedness of physical and emotional well-being. This is not incidental to the work; in many cases, it is the work. As I explore in Part Two of this book, the fascia is the body's quiet, diligent recorder. Intense, unresolved emotions do not simply vanish; they are logged as patterns of physical restriction within the body's connective tissue matrix. When the needle reaches these areas and the tissue releases, the emotional content held within can surface — not because the practitioner has done anything psychological, but because the physical container that was holding the pattern has changed shape.

Fascia-puncture may also contribute to restoring piezoelectric flow within the fascial network. By releasing restrictions, the technique could optimise the flow of bioelectrical signals throughout this interconnected web, potentially enhancing tissue strength, organ function, and promoting a greater sense of overall well-being.

In essence, fascia-puncture transcends the treatment of isolated symptoms. It embodies a holistic approach that acknowledges the interconnectedness of the fascial network and strives to restore its optimal structure and function, ultimately leading to pain relief, improved movement, and enhanced overall health.

Listening With Your Hands

Unlocking the Secrets of Fascia Through Palpation

Skilled palpation is not something that can be fully learned from a textbook. It is developed through thousands of hours of hands-on practice, through the slow accumulation of tactile experience that builds a kind of somatic vocabulary. Each body teaches you something the last body did not. Each restriction has its own character – some feel dense and fibrous, like thickened rope; others feel gluey and reluctant, as though the tissue is stuck to itself; still others feel hot and active, as though an inflammatory process is underway. With time, your hands begin to distinguish not just the physical quality of the tissue but something harder to name – a quality of aliveness or stagnation, of readiness to release or determined holding. These are not mystical perceptions. They are the accumulated pattern recognition of a sensory system that has been trained, over years, to detect very fine differences in tissue quality.

The integration of observation and palpation is essential. A skilled practitioner watches the patient walk into the room, noticing the quality of their gait, the angle of their shoulders, the way they hold their head. This visual information primes the hands – you begin to anticipate where the restrictions might be before you have even touched the skin. Then, when the hands make contact, they confirm or revise these expectations. It is a continuous loop of hypothesis and testing, prediction and correction – not unlike the predictive processing model of the brain itself.

Imagine for a moment that your hands can listen. Not in the way your ears do, but in a deeper, more tactile sense. This is the essence of palpation, a crucial skill in fascia-puncture. Palpation is the art of using your hands to read the story of the body, to feel the subtle textures, tensions, and movements within the fascial network. It is a conversation without words, where your fingertips become detectives, uncovering the clues that guide your treatment.

Developing this sensitivity is like learning a new language. It takes time and practice to discern the difference between smooth, healthy tissue and areas that feel dense, ropy, or even hot. You learn to notice the subtle ways the fascial layers glide over one another, identifying spots where that glide is restricted, indicating adhesions or increased tension. It is like tracing a map of the body's internal landscape, feeling for knots, thickened bands, and points where movement feels stuck.

Often, this listening is combined with watching how someone moves. Seeing how a patient's shoulder struggles to lift can be linked to the tightness you feel along the front, back, or side of their torso. This integration of observation and touch gives you a fuller picture of the functional implications of what you are feeling. And it is not just about the surface; skilled palpation means exploring layer by layer, from the skin to the deeper tissues around muscles and organs. Each layer has its own story to tell, and your hands learn to differentiate them.

To cultivate a refined sense of touch for distinct fascial layers, consider this experiential exercise: place a single strand of hair between two thin sheets of paper. With eyes closed, use your fingertips to locate the hair, relying solely on tactile perception. This hones your ability to differentiate subtle textures and layers, akin to discerning nuances within the fascial system. This hands-on, eyes-closed palpation exercise can be extended into everyday life: while preparing food, consciously feel the varied textures of ingredients; when connecting with nature, take a moment to truly feel the bark of a tree or the texture of leaves, listening with your hands to the tactile information.

For developing an exquisite feel for the fluidity and elasticity of the superficial fascia and skin layers, take two very thin plastic sheets, such as the produce bags found at your local supermarket, and place a tiny amount of mayonnaise between them, creating a synthetic fascial interface. Gently try to move these two layers against each other, observing the resistance and glide. Next, add a tiny bit of water to the mayonnaise and repeat the gliding motion, noting the change in fluidity. Then, add even a little more water and try again. Through this progressive experiment, you will viscerally experience the critical role of hydration in fascial fluidity and the subtle nuances of its elasticity, or the loss thereof.

Mayonnaise and the ground substance found in fascia share striking similarities in their physical properties. Both are viscous fluids. Mayonnaise, an emulsion of oil and water, has a thick, gel-like consistency. Similarly, the ground substance is a hydrated gel containing large molecules like GAGs that give it viscous yet fluid quality. Both serve as lubricants facilitating smooth gliding. The fluidity and lubricating properties of both are highly dependent on water content. In the exercise, adding water changes the consistency, demonstrating improved glide. Similarly, a well-hydrated ground substance is more fluid and elastic, allowing optimal movement. And both serve as a medium – mayonnaise holds ingredients in suspension; the ground substance holds collagen and elastin fibres and allows the exchange of nutrients, waste, and signalling molecules.

Putting the Puzzle Together

The Diagnostic Process

A thorough pre-treatment questionnaire is invaluable. This should inquire about sleep patterns, daytime tiredness, brain fog, past injuries and surgeries, exercise habits, infection susceptibility, digestive disorders, allergies, and current medications. This dual strategy of systematic fascial assessment and thorough patient history not only ensures comprehensive treatment but also significantly conserves valuable time for both the practitioner and the patient.

By knowing which line corresponds to a patient's symptoms, you can target your needling more precisely. If someone has pain along their side, you will pay extra attention to the Lateral Line. While working within these lines, you should keep the myofascial meridians, fascial sequences, or traditional acupuncture meridians in mind. You understand how a restriction in the anterior line might relate to tension in the posterior line or a lateral line.

In practice, you might start by palpating along the anterior line, feeling for tension around the sternum or abdomen. Then, you would move out to the lateral lines, feeling for how the tissue moves and if there are any areas that feel tight or stuck. You would continue this process for each line, always keeping in mind how these lines relate to the patient's specific complaints and to the bigger picture of their overall fascial health.

These vertical lines serve as a tangible and applicable framework, providing a structured approach to delve into the intricate and captivating realm of fascia and its interconnectedness within the human body. They transform the exploration of fascia from an abstract concept to a concrete, map-like system for understanding and addressing movement dysfunctions.

While understanding the web-like nature of fascia is key, sometimes it is helpful to simplify complex anatomical landscapes into more manageable conceptual areas. Imagine consciously dividing the body into systematic vertical lines or zones, much like drawing guiding lines on a canvas. This approach is not about imposing strict, rigid boundaries, but rather offering a practical framework for systematically exploring and treating the body's interconnected fascial system.

The Anterior Line gracefully descends along the very front of your body, extending from below your eyes, down the neck, across the sternum, through the abdomen and pelvis, continuing along the front side of your legs, and ending at the top of your feet.

The Lateral Lines trace paths on either side of the body, stretching from your ears, down the sides of your neck, torso, and legs, to conclude at the sides of your feet.

The Posterior Line originates subtly above your eyebrows, sweeps over your head, follows the full length of your paraspinal muscles, then seamlessly transitions through the gluteal muscles, hamstrings, and calf muscles, before merging into the Achilles tendons and ultimately becoming your plantar fascia, terminating at the bottom of your toes.

The Medial Lines begin at the jaw and anterior neck, intertwine behind the sternum and with the diaphragm, and run from the inner aspect of the low back and abdomen through the pelvis, continuing along the adductor muscles and the deep medial lower legs to the arches of the feet.

The Arm Lines I categorise into Anterior (flexors), Lateral (radial/thumb side), Posterior (extensors), and Medial (ulnar/pinky side) divisions.

These conceptual lines serve as invaluable guides, helping practitioners to systematically navigate the fascial landscape and ensure no significant area is overlooked. By working along these pathways, we can effectively focus attention where it is most needed, guided by the patient's specific complaints and the subtle tactile feedback our hands receive. It is crucial to always remember that these lines are never truly isolated; they are seamlessly interconnected components within the vast, dynamic fascial web.

Fascia-puncture is not just about sticking needles where things feel tight. It is a process of careful investigation, like piecing together a puzzle. We start by listening to the patient's story – when did the pain start? What makes it worse? What is their daily life like? Then we observe, watching them move, how they hold themselves. Palpation is a significant part of it, feeling for clues with our hands. But we also assess movement, checking range of motion, looking for limitations. We need to know about pain patterns – where does it start, and where does it travel? Sometimes, we might need additional tests to rule out other issues. And we cannot ignore the emotional side of things – sometimes, feelings are tied up in that tension.

When rotational movements are limited, restrictions affecting external rotation are often localised around the convergence point of the posterior and lateral lines. Conversely, limitations associated with internal rotation can frequently be traced to the intersection of the anterior and lateral lines. Understanding these anatomical relationships allows for a more targeted approach to assessment and treatment, focusing on releasing tension and restoring optimal movement patterns.

The Treatment

Transforming Health from Within

The light rotation applied to the needle after insertion is a key element. This gentle manipulation engages the collagen fibres within the fascia, creating a subtle mechanical stretch and promoting relaxation of the surrounding tissues. The sensation of spaghetti around the fork suggests a gentle winding of the fibres, which could help to release cross-links and improve glide.

The occasional sensation of an electric twitch indicates a direct stimulation of the local myofascia. This involuntary muscle contraction followed by relaxation can be a powerful mechanism for releasing tension and reducing pressure on nerve endings. It suggests an interaction with the neuromuscular system within the fascial environment. This phenomenon is often perceived as a brief, tingling or jumping sensation by the patient, and it is generally a positive sign, indicating that the needle has contacted a reactive area within the tissue. It is important to communicate this potential sensation to the patient beforehand so they are not surprised or alarmed.

Post-treatment sensation deserves attention. It is important to inform patients that they might experience some local soreness or a feeling of mild aching in the treated area after the needles are removed. This is a normal response, akin to the muscle soreness one might feel after exercise, and it typically subsides within a day or two. Advising them to stay hydrated and to avoid strenuous activity immediately following treatment can help minimise post-treatment discomfort. In some cases, patients might also experience a sense of relaxation or even a slight fatigue after the session, as the body begins to integrate the changes from the treatment.

By integrating these nuanced aspects of needle selection, insertion, manipulation, and post-treatment care, fascia-puncture becomes a highly skilled and patient-centred practice, going beyond mere needle placement to truly engage with the body's complex fascial network. It is a process of listening, responding, and gently guiding the tissue towards a state of greater balance and ease.

Fascia-puncture excels in treating musculoskeletal pain, including persistent issues like low back pain, stiff neck and shoulders, and headaches. It can also address tendonitis resulting from sports or repetitive actions, as fascial tension frequently contributes to these conditions. We might find restrictions in the posterior lines, or tightness in the front of the neck. By releasing these areas, we can bring relief. It is about finding those restrictions in the body and gently letting them go.

Yet it is not just about pain; it is about movement. After surgery, scar tissue can limit mobility. Injuries can leave us feeling stuck. Even simple stiffness can hold us back. Fascia-puncture can help break up adhesions, soften scar tissue, and restore that sense of freedom. It is useful for frozen shoulders, sports injuries, and anything that is hindering the way we move.

We cannot ignore that our bodies hold more than just muscles and bones. Our emotions can get tangled up in our tissues, manifesting as tension. And releasing that tension can bring emotional release too. Sometimes, patients might cry or feel a wave of relief washing over them. It is about creating a safe space for that to happen, acknowledging that healing is not just physical.

Safety first: when engaging in therapeutic interventions that involve needling, paramount importance must be placed on safety and adherence to best practices. This commitment begins with rigorous hygiene protocols – ensuring the sterility of all needles, preparing or cleaning the patient's skin, and maintaining an impeccably tidy and disinfected treatment area are absolute non-negotiables. These measures are fundamental in preventing infection and safeguarding patient well-being.

Equally vital is a profound and comprehensive understanding of human anatomy. Practitioners must possess in-depth knowledge of the underlying structures to meticulously avoid vital areas such as major blood vessels, nerves, and organs like the lungs. This anatomical precision is particularly crucial when treating more delicate patients, such as those who are very thin or fragile, where the margin for error is significantly reduced.

Beyond the technical aspects, clear and empathetic communication with the patient is paramount. Before any intervention, it is essential to thoroughly explain what they can expect during the procedure, address any concerns, and answer all their questions. This fosters trust and ensures a comfortable, informed experience. Providing explicit post-treatment guidance on self-care is crucial for supporting the healing process.

Central to the efficacy of fascia-puncture is the refined skill of palpation. Our hands become our primary diagnostic tool, allowing us to perceive subtle yet significant nuances within the fascial web. During palpation, we are meticulously assessing for increased tension, restricted gliding ability, altered tissue elasticity, puffy or oedematous skin, localised areas that are unusually cold or warm, and even distinct variations in skin colour or surface texture. Each of these findings can indicate an underlying fascial restriction, suggesting a potential point for intervention. This granular sensitivity implies that virtually any square-millimetre of the body can become a potential fascia-puncture point, provided it correlates with palpable dysfunction. Our ability to meticulously adjust the angle of needle insertion further enhances precision.

In my practice, I primarily use 0.3mm thin and 25mm long single-use acupuncture needles, a safe length that aligns with palpable tissue depth. While I avoid longer needles, skilled practitioners may use them. For hands, feet, and the face, I utilise shorter, 0.16mm thin and 8mm Koryo Sooji Chim needles. Insertion is performed gently and accurately. A guide tube assists with the 25mm needles, and a special injector is used for the 8mm needles. The needle is typically inserted 0.5 to 2.5cm deep, targeting the deep fascia, intermuscular spaces, tendons, ligaments, or joint structures. Inserting beyond 1 to 2cm offers minimal additional benefit for connective tissue stretching, as the strong fibrous layers are located more superficially.

Then comes the spaghetti around the fork – a gentle unilateral rotation of the needle to engage collagen fibres, winding them up and stretching them. Sometimes, you will feel an electric twitch, a sign that you have hit a spot that needs releasing. Needles stay in for a while, allowing the body to respond, and then they are gently removed. During the removal, one can observe and feel the decompression of the connective tissue as the thick fascial layers wrap around it, resulting in a visible stretch and lifting of both skin and fascia.

In my practice, the number of needles per session is directly correlated with the complexity and extent of fascial restrictions. For localised issues, such as specific elbow tendonitis, a typical session might involve 20 to 30 needles. However, for chronic back pain with numerous underlying restrictions, sessions frequently necessitate 40 to 60 or even more needles.

A particularly insightful aspect of palpation during a session involves observing the movement of previously inserted needles. As we palpate surrounding fascial regions, we use the needle's response as a dynamic diagnostic tool. With experience, we can discern whether a needle inserted in the distal IT-band moves more or less than expected when pressure is applied around the proximal IT-band origin. This subtle feedback provides real-time information about fascial interconnectedness.

In the practice of fascia-puncture as outlined in this book, electro-acupuncture is intentionally not utilised. This choice is rooted in several considerations. The scientific principles underlying fascia-puncture revolve around eliciting a specific connective tissue wind-up around the needle, which facilitates fascial release.

This intricate mechanical and cellular response relies on the body's own bioelectrical currents and precise mechanical manipulation, without requiring external electrical current. The nature of therapeutically applied external current differs significantly from the subtle piezoelectric currents naturally produced within collagen fibres. Clinical comparisons have shown that while comparable pain relief might be achieved with electro-acupuncture, it often shows lesser improvement in other symptoms such as anxiety or pain avoidance behaviour. This discrepancy is most likely due to a hypothesised blockage of ascending information at the spinal cord level, which may prevent a complete range of signals from reaching the brain, reducing the holistic homeostatic response. Instead, fascia-puncture prioritises the gentle yet profoundly effective unilateral rotational stimulation, encouraging a more integrated and natural healing response.

The gentle manipulation of the needle after insertion is key. The sensation of spaghetti around the fork suggests a gentle winding of the fibres, which helps release cross-links and improve glide. The occasional electric twitch indicates direct stimulation of local myofascia. This involuntary contraction followed by relaxation is a powerful mechanism for releasing tension. It is important to communicate this potential sensation to the patient beforehand.

Retention times typically range from 15 minutes to 30 minutes. During this time, the gentle mechanical stimulation and the body's physiological responses continue to work on releasing fascial restrictions. Needle withdrawal should be smooth and controlled, with gentle pressure applied to the puncture site. Post-withdrawal palpation reassesses changes in tissue texture.

Throughout the procedure, maintain open communication with the patient. Each individual is unique, and tailoring the treatment to their specific needs is essential. Patients may experience some local soreness or mild aching after treatment, typically subsiding within a day or two. Advise hydration and avoidance of strenuous activity immediately following treatment.

Contraindications

Needles can cause bleeding, and in individuals with certain blood clotting disorders or strong blood-thinning medication, even a small puncture could lead to prolonged bleeding or bruising. It is like navigating a boat in stormy waters – the risk is much higher.

In situations like acute trauma, severe infections, or other serious medical crises, fascia-puncture is simply not the right approach. The priority is addressing the emergency. Pregnancy is a special time with its own set of considerations. While fascia-puncture might be appropriate in some cases and with specific training, certain areas and trimesters are considered contraindications. Always err on the side of caution.

Then there are relative contraindications, where we need to proceed with extra care. If someone's immune system is weakened, they are more susceptible to infection. We need to be extra diligent with hygiene and possibly adjust our needle depth or technique. Severe systemic diseases – conditions like cancer, autoimmune disorders, or other serious illnesses – require careful consideration of the potential impact of fascia-puncture. Special care is needed for recent surgery, fresh wounds, or fractures. We may avoid direct treatment in the acute healing phase and wait until the tissue has stabilised.

Fear of needles is common. We need to be patient, explain the process clearly, and use techniques like guide tubes to make the experience as comfortable as possible. It is about building trust and easing anxieties. Lymphoedema and other swellings involving fluid buildup due to a compromised lymphatic system require mindfulness of needle placement, avoiding areas where lymph nodes are concentrated.

Releasing the Restrictions

Addressing Common Musculoskeletal Pain

Musculoskeletal pain is something many of us encounter. Whether it is a persistent ache, a sudden sharp pain, or a nagging stiffness, these discomforts can seriously affect daily lives. Fascia-puncture can often provide significant relief by addressing the fascial restrictions that contribute to these issues.

It is crucial to remember that our muscles and bones do not work in isolation. They are all intricately connected through the fascial web. When fascia becomes tight, restricted, or adhered, it can pull on muscles, compress nerves, and limit joint movement, leading to pain.

Low back pain, one of the most prevalent complaints, frequently finds its roots in fascial restrictions. We often discover significant tightness within the Posterior Line, which spans from the feet all the way up the back, over the head, to the top of your eyebrows. This means that a seemingly localised issue, such as persistent calf muscle tightness, can alter the entire biomechanical tension of this posterior chain, leading to increased pressure on the low back. In such cases, carefully needling the calves can bring additional and often profound benefits beyond just using local needles in the lumbar region. Beyond the Posterior Line itself, the thoracolumbar fascia and the quadratus lumborum muscles are frequently found to hold significant tension. Restrictions in the Anterior Line, Lateral Lines, or External Rotation Line can all indirectly increase tension and contribute to lumbar discomfort. And of course, we must never overlook the emotional dimension; chronic back pain often carries a significant emotional component, with stress, anxiety, and unresolved emotional tensions frequently manifesting as persistent fascial tightening in the lumbar region.

Neck and shoulder pain frequently stems from or is influenced by fascial restrictions. Tension in the Anterior Line can exert a pulling force on the neck and shoulders. The upper trapezius muscles often become excessively tight, as do the scalene muscles. Localised knots known as trigger points can develop, referring pain to the head, arms, and upper back. Crucially, what presents as neck or shoulder pain might be a compensatory pattern stemming from a seemingly unrelated issue elsewhere – for example, an old ankle injury altering fascial tension and biomechanics of the entire leg, pelvis, and spine.

Headaches are a common ailment that you might not immediately connect with fascial health, yet restrictions in the neck, jaw, and scalp muscles can be a major contributing source. Tension headaches are frequently driven by localised fascial tightness. Cervicogenic headaches originating in the neck are another type where releasing tension can be a game-changer. Distant restrictions in the lower or upper leg can subtly alter the entire fascial web's tension patterns, increasing pressure in the cervical region and potentially decreasing blood flow to the head. Dehydration, nutritional sensitivities, and systemic inflammation are also important considerations.

Myofascial Pain Syndrome represents a chronic and often debilitating condition characterised by trigger points in multiple muscles and their surrounding fascia, leading to widespread referred pain. Fascia-puncture, combined with stretching and myofascial release, can be remarkably effective. In some individuals, genetic collagen fibre disorders can impact the inherent properties of fascial tissue, making it less resilient or slower to respond. In such cases, the long-term aim often shifts from a complete cure to managing the condition to a bearable state.

Tendonitis, whether in the wrist, elbow, ankles, or other regions, involves not just inflammation of the tendon itself but reduced gliding of tendon sheaths with the surrounding fascia. Treatment must follow the myofascial connections beyond the immediate pain area. For medial epicondylitis, one would focus on the medial/ulnar side from wrist through elbow to the posterior-medial shoulder. For lateral epicondylitis, the focus shifts to the radial side extending past the biceps toward the deltoid. Similarly, ankle tendonitis often requires attention to the lateral line.

Plantar fasciitis, a common and debilitating foot pain affecting the plantar fascia, typically manifests as sharp pain in the heel. Fascia-puncture can be highly effective in releasing tension and improving flexibility. The Medial Line plays an indispensable role in building and maintaining the foot's arch. A compromised Medial Line places excessive strain on the plantar fascia.

In each of these conditions, fascia-puncture works by directly addressing underlying fascial restrictions. Fine needles are inserted into areas of palpable tension and altered glide. The gentle manipulation initiates a cascade of therapeutic effects: breaking down collagen cross-links, releasing adhesions, improving mobility and glide, modulating pain signals, enhancing blood flow and hydration, and triggering natural healing mechanisms.

Restoring Movement

Enhancing Mobility and Function

Beyond simply alleviating pain, fascia-puncture holds immense potential for restoring movement and enhancing function. When our movement is restricted due to fascial adhesions, scar tissue, or chronic tension, it can feel like we are trapped in a body that does not quite belong to us. The joy of moving freely, of exploring the world without limitations, becomes dimmed. Fascia-puncture offers a pathway to reclaim that sense of freedom.

Post-surgical rehabilitation is a significant area where fascia-puncture excels. Surgery inevitably involves cutting through tissues, including fascia. Scar tissue can become excessive or disorganised, creating adhesions that bind tissues together. Fascia-puncture, when integrated into a rehabilitation programme, can gently break down these adhesions, softening scar tissue and restoring natural glide. It is like unzipping a stuck zipper.

Sports injuries push the body to its limits. Injuries cause inflammation and fascial restrictions. Muscle imbalances develop as the body tries to protect an injured area. These restrictions impede performance and increase the risk of future injuries. Fascia-puncture can address these imbalances by releasing tight spots, improving flexibility, and enhancing movement patterns. It is about fine-tuning the instrument so it plays in perfect harmony.

Frozen shoulder, or adhesive capsulitis, is characterised by stiffness and pain that often develops slowly and significantly restricts arm movement. Inflammation and thickening of the shoulder joint capsule and surrounding fascia play a significant role. Fascia-puncture, combined with gentle movement therapy and stretching, can help stretch and release these restricted tissues, gradually restoring mobility.

Scar tissue management extends beyond post-surgical scars. Scar tissue from various injuries is denser and less elastic than normal tissue, and it can adhere to surrounding structures. Fascia-puncture can help soften and release scar tissue, making it more pliable and reducing its restrictive effects.

Restoring the Flow

Beyond Mechanical Release

While fascia-puncture certainly has a mechanical effect on tissues, its benefits extend beyond just the physical. When movement is restored, it can have a profound impact on other aspects of well-being.

Improved proprioception comes with increased movement. The body receives more sensory input, enhancing our sense of where we are in space. This improved awareness leads to better coordination, balance, and a greater sense of embodiment. Increased circulation follows naturally — movement is essential for healthy circulation, bringing vital nutrients and oxygen while removing waste products.

Emotional well-being is intrinsically linked to movement. When we move freely, we feel more alive and connected to our bodies. When movement is restricted, we may feel trapped and disconnected. Restoring movement often leads to emotional release and improved mood. Ultimately, restoring movement significantly enhances quality of life. When we can move without pain or restriction, we can participate more fully in the activities we enjoy.

Beyond its documented impact on musculoskeletal pain and movement, the improvement of fascial gliding and the release of fascial restrictions profoundly enhance the workings of internal organs. Our organs are enveloped by and suspended within visceral fascia, which is inextricably linked to the broader musculoskeletal fascial web. When restrictions in the surrounding fascia are released, it can reduce extrinsic pressure on organs, optimise their motility, and improve local blood flow and nerve supply. Consequently, fascia-puncture can offer significant support to patients with conditions such as gastro-oesophageal reflux disease, various digestive disorders, and potentially improve fertility by optimising the environment and mobility of reproductive organs. This holistic effect underscores fascia's crucial role as a unifying system that influences not just movement, but the vital functions of our internal physiology.

In essence, fascia-puncture is not solely about addressing pain; it is about unlocking the body's innate potential for movement, vitality, and full participation in life. By freeing the fascial web, we liberate the body, allowing it to flow, explore, and express itself with greater ease and grace.

Quieting the Monkey

The Practice of Living in the Territory

Part II built the case for how the Monkey constructs its world. This is where we find out what to actually do with it.

What Part III offers is a set of graduated practices for loosening the Monkey's grip. Not for silencing it – the attempt to silence the Monkey produces its own distortions, its own subtle cages. For creating the conditions under which the silence that already exists between the Monkey's sentences becomes more available, more familiar, more inhabitable. Begin wherever you are drawn. Return to what genuinely opens something in you.

If the earlier chapters built the map, what follows now moves more fully into the territory. The question is no longer only what the

Storytelling Monkey does, but what becomes possible when its activity is seen clearly.

The Monkey, at this stage of the book, has a particularly subtle strategy: it will begin to read the practices as a project. A goal. A measure of progress toward a destination. Notice this. Set it gently aside. The practices are not a path to the territory. They are a way of removing what has been preventing the territory from being noticed.

These practices are not arbitrary. Each one targets a specific lever that the neuroscience identified. Breath work reaches the autonomic nervous system through the vagus nerve, shifting the body's predictive baseline from threat to safety. Somatic attention generates new proprioceptive signals that give the brain's prediction engine something more current to update toward. Un-Naming disrupts the narrative priors that the Monkey uses to foreclose on experience before it arrives. These are not meditations on calming down. They are precision interventions in the mechanism Part II described. The science pointed at them. The practices are what the science was pointing at.

The following chapters are adapted from The Storytelling Monkey: Where Neuroscience ends and Wisdom begins.

Coming Home to the Body

"All things flourish and go back to where they started. Going back is stillness. Stillness is what is. Knowing what is – clarity."

– Daodejing, Chapter 16

Proprioception, the Web of Life, and the Pre-Narrative Now

The body's report is already running. Before the first sentence of any story, before the Monkey can narrate what is happening, the happening is already in progress – in the tissue, in the fluid, in the ceaseless transmission of information about where the organism is, how it is positioned, what is happening inside it at this precise moment. This report requires no language. It requires no Storyteller to receive it. It is the organism in direct, unmediated conversation with itself. This is proprioception.

And it is the most reliable entry point back to the territory beneath the map.

The Monkey filters this proprioceptive information through its model. What it hands you is a simplified summary of the body – efficient enough for navigation, edited well below the body's actual resolution. The raw signal was never interrupted. The practice of returning attention to sensation is not mysticism. It is the recovery of data the Monkey has been editing for efficiency's sake. The data was always there.

The body's self-sensing apparatus includes mechanoreceptors distributed throughout the fascial web – sensors embedded in the connective tissue that respond to pressure, stretch, vibration, and fluid movement. It includes the interoceptive system: the sensing of the body's internal state through heartbeat, temperature, digestion, the quality of each breath. It includes the vestibular system in the inner ear, tracking orientation and movement in space. Taken together, these constitute the body's pre-narrative report of the present moment. Before the Monkey can tell you what you are feeling, or what it means, or what you should do about it – this system is already reporting, with far greater fidelity than conscious narrative and without editorial comment, the organism's present condition.

Fascia is a major contributor to proprioceptive signalling and one of the body's most important sensory tissues, though not the only pathway through which proprioceptive information is generated and processed. The fascial web is extraordinarily densely innervated, described by some researchers as among the richest sensory tissues in the body, though comparative claims remain an active area of fascial research. What is not in doubt is its functional centrality: fascia is a critical intermediary in how the body senses and reports its own condition. A restriction in the plantar fascia of the right foot generates a tensional adjustment that travels up the posterior chain, affects the position of the sacrum, alters the mechanics of the breathing diaphragm, and influences the fascial tension around the skull. The web does not narrate. It transmits. And in that transmission, every part of the organism is continuously in conversation with every other part.

The Practice of Proprioceptive Listening

Here is where I am going to ask you to stop reading for a moment. Until now, you have almost certainly not felt your clothes since you put them on this morning. Feel them now. The weight of fabric on your shoulders. The texture against the skin of your forearms. The slight pressure of a collar or a waistband or socks against the skin. These sensations have been present every moment since you dressed. The Monkey simply had more interesting things to narrate, and so it filtered them out. They were available the entire time. The territory was always there.

Turn the attention inward now. Find your heartbeat — not as a concept, but as a physical event happening in the body. Where can you detect it? The chest is the obvious place, but the heartbeat is present throughout the vascular system. Can you feel it in the neck? In the wrists? In the temples, or the soles of the feet? Follow it from the heart outward – downward through the abdomen, the pelvis, the legs, to the feet and toes. This takes patience. The Monkey will want to narrate the search. Acknowledge that, and return to the actual physical pulse: the slight, rhythmic pressure that moves through the body thirty thousand times a day without your permission or direction.

The practice extends naturally into movement. Walking barefoot – actually attending to the sensory information arriving from the soles of the feet with each step – is one of the most direct and accessible forms of proprioceptive training available. The plantar surface of the foot is among the most densely innervated areas of the body. The fascial web of the sole connects directly to the Superficial Back Line that runs upward through the entire posterior chain. What the feet report about the ground shapes the tension pattern of the whole body. When we disconnect the feet from their sensory environment inside shoes, we are disconnecting the body's most fundamental point of contact with the earth it stands on. Every barefoot step, attended to honestly, is a small return to the territory.

The final and most important dimension of proprioceptive practice is what happens with language when sensation is encountered. When attention rests on a sensation and a label arrives – my back hurts again, my knee is tight, I'm tired – the label immediately narrows and files the encounter. The Monkey has what it needs. It moves on. The practice is to replace the storied, personal label with something more descriptive and less identified. Not my back hurts again – which incorporates the sensation into a history, a self-concept, an expectation about what this means – but there is an ache in the lower lumbar region. Not I am exhausted – but there is a quality of heaviness in the limbs and a particular slowness in the breath. This is a structural shift in how the nervous system relates to what it is experiencing. The personal label activates the

Default Mode Network; it becomes part of the Monkey's ongoing story about who you are and what your body is like. The descriptive observation keeps the experience in the present tense, in the body, in the territory. It remains alive rather than filed.

What the body knew:

The fascial web was present before the Storytelling Monkey arrived, and it will continue its quiet conversation long after every particular story has dissolved. Proprioception is not a technique – it is the recovery of the organism's most original mode of knowing. The body does not ask what anything means. It simply reports what is. In that report – heard without interpretation, met without judgement, attended to with the patient curiosity of someone arriving home – the territory reveals itself exactly as it is.

Breathing as the Bridge

"Can you concentrate your breath and become as soft as an infant?"

– Daodejing, Chapter 10

The One Autonomic Function You Can Control – and Why That Changes Everything

Every entry point into the territory beneath the map requires something of you before you arrive. Proprioception requires you to know enough about the body to listen to it. Un-Naming requires familiarity with the gap between sensation and label. The practices in Chapter 14 require a degree of autonomic stability that most modern bodies do not begin with. The breath requires nothing. You already have it. It has been running since the moment you were born, without your permission or awareness, and it is running right now. The question is only whether you are going to participate in it consciously, or continue to let it run on the Monkey's autopilot.

The breath is the single point of structural overlap between the voluntary and involuntary nervous systems. Every other process the Monkey runs on — the heartbeat, the hormonal cascade, the fascial contraction in response to perceived threat — happens without your conscious access. You cannot decide to slow your heart rate the way you can decide to slow your breathing. You cannot instruct your psoas to release the way you can instruct your hand to open. But you can choose to breathe differently. And because the breath is the point of overlap, that choice propagates outward into every system the will cannot otherwise reach. This is anatomy. And it means that the simplest available act of attention — a slow, nasal, diaphragmatic breath — is a direct intervention in the biological substrate of the Monkey's narrative.

Polyvagal Theory: Why Felt Safety Is the First Practice

Polyvagal Theory describes the body's system for assessing safety before the

Monkey can form a single word about it. We need it in full here – because understanding why the breath works requires understanding what it is actually crossing.

Porges, a distinguished professor of psychiatry at the University of North Carolina, developed the theory over several decades of research into the autonomic nervous system and its role in social behaviour, emotional regulation, and health. The name comes from the vagus nerve – the tenth cranial nerve, the great wandering nerve that connects the brainstem to almost every major organ – and from its polyvagal, or multi-branched, structure. What Porges revealed is that the vagus nerve is not a single system but two: a phylogenetically older, unmyelinated branch and a newer, myelinated one. These two branches do not simply do more or less of the same job. They do categorically different jobs, and they activate in a hierarchical sequence that the theory describes with great precision.

Three States, Three Bodies

Porges describes three broad states of autonomic organisation, each associated with a distinct evolutionary heritage and a distinct pattern of physiological, emotional, and social experience.

The ventral vagal state is the most recently evolved. Associated with the myelinated branch of the vagus – the 'smart vagus' – it is the biological substrate of what we recognise as normal social engagement. When the ventral vagal system is active, the organism is in a state of genuine safety. The middle ear muscles are tuned to the frequency range of the human voice. The face is animated, expressive, receptive. The heart rate is variable and flexible. Breathing is full and rhythmic. The muscles of the neck and head support an upright, open posture. The organism is, in the physiological sense, available: available to connection, available to learning, available to the quality of genuine presence that the practices in this book are attempting to cultivate.

The sympathetic activation state is older. It is the state of mobilisation – fight or flight, preparation for action against threat. When the nervous system's pre-conscious assessment – what Porges calls neuroception – detects cues of danger, the sympathetic system overrides the ventral vagal. The heart accelerates. The breath shortens and rises into the chest. The muscles of the trunk brace. The middle ear tunes away from the human voice and toward the lower frequencies that, in evolutionary history, signalled large predators. The face flattens. Social engagement becomes literally neurologically inaccessible – not as a choice, but as the direct consequence of a state change that did not ask the Monkey's opinion.

The dorsal vagal state is the oldest. Associated with the unmyelinated branch of the vagus – the primitive, reptilian branch – it is the state of last resort when threat is overwhelming and fight or flight has failed. Shutdown. Freeze. The collapse of organismic energy that we recognise clinically as dissociation, numbness, and the particular absence of presence that characterises severe depression and unresolved trauma. The heart rate drops. The breath becomes shallow. The body stills. In the evolutionary context of an organism caught by a predator, playing dead is a survival strategy. In the context of a human being living inside a story of unresolvable threat, it is the physiological substrate of despair.

These three states are not personality types, and they are not choices. They are biological configurations that the nervous system moves between in response to neuroceptive assessment — an assessment that operates below conscious awareness and that the Monkey subsequently narrates as emotion, mood, and character. The person who has spent years in chronic sympathetic activation is not anxious by nature. They are physiologically organised for threat. The person who has moved into dorsal shutdown is not lacking willpower. They are in a state the nervous system selected as the least costly available response to an experience of unresolvable overwhelm. This changes the entire moral architecture of how we understand human behaviour.

The Vagal Brake: What the Breath Actually Moves

The physiological mechanism that connects conscious breath practice to this three-state system is what Porges calls the vagal brake. The myelinated vagus, when it is well-toned and active, exerts a continuous inhibitory influence on the heart – slowing it below its intrinsic pacemaker rate. This inhibition is the vagal brake. It is what allows the healthy organism to maintain a resting heart rate well below the natural baseline of approximately one hundred beats per minute. A well-toned vagal brake is the physiological signature of the ventral vagal state – of felt safety, of flexibility, of the organism's capacity to engage without defensiveness.

When neuroception detects danger, the vagal brake is released – the inhibition lifts – and the heart accelerates into sympathetic activation. When the threat exceeds the sympathetic system's capacity, the dorsal vagal overrides entirely. The movement between states corresponds to the sequential engagement and release of these two vagal branches, operating in a hierarchy that Porges calls the polyvagal ladder. The organism moves up and down the ladder in continuous response to the assessment of environmental safety.

The reason conscious breathing practice works – the reason it works with a precision that no cognitive intervention can match – is that the breath is the one lever the voluntary nervous system has direct access to inside this hierarchy. Slow, controlled, nasal breathing tones the vagal brake directly. The baroreceptors in the aorta and carotid arteries, which monitor blood pressure, communicate with the vagus nerve in a rhythm that is maximally synchronised at approximately six breath cycles per minute – the resonance frequency of the cardiovascular system. Every slow, full breath cycle is a direct input to the neuroceptive system: safety is available here. The brake can engage. Every patient who arrives in chronic sympathetic activation – shoulders elevated, jaw set, breath short and high – is in a nervous system state that forecloses the very openness that healing requires. The state must shift first. The breath is the fastest, most reliable, most accessible way to shift it.

Felt Safety Is Not a Feeling

Porges makes a distinction that I want to press on, because it is clinically indispensable. Felt safety – the physiological condition of the ventral vagal state – is not the same as the cognitive assessment of safety. A patient can know, rationally and in complete intellectual honesty, that they are in no danger on the treatment table. They can say so, mean it, and believe it. And still present with the autonomic signature of threat. Because neuroception is not reading the Monkey's narrative. It is reading the cues in the environment: the quality of the light, the tone of my voice, the micro-expressions in my face, the postural signals of nearby bodies, the proprioceptive input from their own tissue about its current state of tension.

If those cues carry the residue of past threat – if the smell of a clinical environment, or the quality of a stranger's hands on their body, has been conditioned by previous experience to signal danger – the neuroceptive system will respond to what it detects, not to what the patient consciously believes.

This is why establishing physiological safety – ventral vagal engagement – before any other clinical intervention is not merely good therapeutic practice. It is a necessary biological prerequisite. I spend considerable time at the beginning of every session attending to the patient's autonomic state before I attend to their tissue. The quality of my voice, the pace of my movements, the degree of physical contact I initiate before the patient has had time to register safety – all of this is an attempt to support the upregulation of the ventral vagal system. To give the neuroceptive assessment enough genuine cues of safety that the vagal brake can engage and the tissue can become available.

Porges' framework also suggests something beyond the mechanics of breath: the quality of the environment in which breathing happens matters. The neuroceptive system is reading everything. A meditation practice undertaken in a room made carefully to feel safe will support ventral vagal engagement more effectively than the same practice in a noisy, unpredictable environment. This is not over-sensitivity. It is how the nervous system was built. We are a profoundly social species, and our biology of felt safety is fundamentally interpersonal – designed to be co-regulated, to read cues from nearby bodies, to settle in the presence of other settled nervous systems. Practising with others has a biological logic that practising alone does not fully replicate.

Light, Slow, Deep: The Three Principles of Functional Breathing

When the vagus nerve is suppressed – as it is under chronic stress, in trauma states, and in many of the patients who find their way to my table – the organism lives in chronic activation that the Monkey happily narrates as personality: I am an anxious person. I have never been able to relax. Slow, nasal, diaphragmatic breathing is the most direct available stimulus to change this.

In my work I use the framework I call LSD: Light, Slow, Deep. Three words that carry considerably more precision than they appear to.

Light means silent. Breathing so gently that a feather placed beneath the nose would barely stir. This is not atmospheric – it is physiological. Gentle breathing allows a slight, healthy accumulation of carbon dioxide in the bloodstream. Most people believe more oxygen is always better. In fact, what the Bohr effect demonstrates is that oxygen delivery to the tissues depends not on the concentration of oxygen in the blood but on the balance between oxygen and carbon dioxide: haemoglobin releases oxygen to the tissues more readily in the presence of CO2. Breathing too much – even mildly and chronically, as many people do under sustained stress – reduces CO2, constricts blood vessels, and paradoxically reduces tissue oxygenation. Light breathing optimises this balance. It makes the oxygen you already have more available.

Slow means approximately six breaths per minute – five seconds in, five seconds out. This is the cardiovascular resonance frequency: the rhythm at which heart rate variability is maximised and the nervous and cardiovascular systems synchronise most efficiently. High HRV is associated with resilience, emotional regulation, and cognitive flexibility. Low HRV – which accompanies chronic stress and the chronic fascial tension that goes with it – is associated with rigidity, reactivity, and the kind of fixed narrative identity the Monkey mistakes for a permanent Self. Slow breathing is, in the most precise neurological sense, the practice of flexibility.

Deep means directed downward into the belly, through the full descent of the diaphragm. The diaphragm is not merely a breathing muscle. It is the roof of the body's core canister, intimately connected through fascial continuity to the pelvic floor below, the deep spinal muscles behind, and the transversus abdominis in front. It shares critical fascial connections with the psoas — the deep hip flexor that is, in my clinical experience, one of the most consistently overloaded structures in the body of a chronically stressed modern human. When the diaphragm moves freely, it creates a rhythmic internal massage of the surrounding connective tissues, stimulates the vagus nerve directly, and hydrates the fascial web through the gentle pumping action of alternating pressure. Deep breathing, done correctly, is the most accessible form of self-myofascial release available. It can happen at any moment of any day.

PRACTICE: *The 5:5 Foundation Practice*

Find a comfortable position, seated or lying down. Allow the eyes to close. Place one hand on the chest and one on the lower belly. Your goal: the belly hand moves; the chest hand stays still.

Close the mouth gently. Rest the tongue against the roof of the mouth. Inhale slowly and lightly through the nose for a count of 5 seconds, allowing the belly to expand. Exhale slowly and completely through the nose for a count of 5 seconds, allowing the belly to soften.

Continue for a minimum of 10 minutes. Twice daily if possible. When the Monkey intervenes with commentary, planning, or judgement – notice it, without engagement, and return to the count. The return is the practice. The noticing is the practice. The counting is only the scaffold.

Simple breathing rhythms can be practised without making them complicated. Six breaths per minute is often a useful resting rhythm. You can approach this through five seconds in and ten seconds out, and in longer practice sessions some people respond well to a still longer exhale – fifteen or even twenty seconds – provided the breath remains light and unforced. Two other accessible patterns are box breathing (four seconds in, four seconds hold, four seconds out, four seconds hold) and the well-known 4-7-8 rhythm. The ratio matters less than the quality of the breath and the body's response to it.

A patient I will call Teresa, in her mid-fifties, presented with hypertension following a vaccination a few back. She had been hypotonic throughout most of her life. After the vaccination, however, she began to experience very high blood-pressure readings, often with systolic values between 150 and 180. At one recent doctor's visit, her initial reading was around 160/110. She then used a simple breathing rhythm we had discussed: five seconds inhaling through the nose, followed by ten seconds exhaling. Within minutes, the second measurement had returned to a normal range. The point is not that breath solves every hypertensive presentation. It is that breathing can, in some cases, alter functions of the body that otherwise appear beyond voluntary influence.

What the body knew:

The breath is not a relaxation technique. It is a direct intervention in the biological systems that the Storytelling Monkey's narrative runs on. Every slow, nasal, diaphragmatic breath is a signal to the vagus nerve that safety is available. Every moment of conscious breathing is a choice to participate in the organism's own healing capacity — to step, briefly and deliberately, out of the Monkey's story and into the body that has never left.

Un-Naming

"The form of the formless, the image of the imageless. Call it elusive. Meet it and you cannot see its face. Follow it and you cannot see its back."

— Daodejing, Chapter 8

The Practice of Seeing Without Labels

Earlier in this book, we traced how naming operates at the level of tissue: the label becomes the story, the story becomes the restriction, the restriction becomes the person. Un-Naming is the practice of reversing this sequence – not by arguing with the label, but by attending, with genuine curiosity, to what was present before the label arrived. The sensation, encountered directly, is almost always more dynamic, more specific, and more changeable than the story about it.

Starting With Sensation

The most accessible entry point for Un-Naming is physical sensation. Consider pain. Pain is one of the Monkey's most elaborately labelled experiences. My bad knee. My old shoulder injury. My chronic back. Each label carries an entire architecture of story – a history, a prognosis, an identity, a set of expectations about what is possible and what is not. The label arrives with the sensation, and by the time the person is consciously aware of their bad knee, they are not actually encountering their knee. They are encountering the story of their knee, which is considerably more fixed and considerably less interesting than the actual, living, dynamic tissue that is doing something real and present in this moment.

Try this now. Bring attention to any area of physical discomfort or tension in your body. Let the label come – whatever the Monkey offers. Then, gently, set the label to one side. Not deny it. Not argue with it. Move it aside the way you might move a newspaper off a table to see what is underneath. And look at what is actually there. Is it pressure? Heat? A quality of vibration? Is there pulsing, or stillness? Is it constant, or does it shift? Is it sharp or diffuse? Is there a direction to it? How large is it, and where exactly are its edges?

These are not the questions of a medical diagnosis. They are the questions of direct encounter. And what almost always happens when people practise this is that the sensation changes. Not always immediately, and not always dramatically. But the relationship to it changes. The story of a permanent, fixed, chronic condition loosens slightly when the condition is encountered directly rather than through its label. The territory turns out to be more dynamic, more responsive, and more interesting than the map had insisted.

Un-Naming Emotion

The same practice applied to emotional states is simultaneously more challenging and more revealing. I am angry. I am anxious. I am sad. Each statement collapses a complex, shifting, embodied state into a single word — and then, critically, incorporates it into identity. The emotion has become the Self. Un-Naming emotion does not mean denying or suppressing it. It means meeting it with the same quality of direct attention that we bring to physical sensation. Where in the body is it? What is its texture? What is its quality as a physical experience, before the Monkey supplies the name?

This is not a technique for emotional avoidance. It is a technique for deeper emotional contact. When I label a state as anxiety and then try to manage the label, I am managing a concept. When I follow the physical reality of the state – the tightening across the chest, the contraction in the belly, the slight holding of breath, the restless quality of the hands – I am in contact with the actual experience. And from that contact, something that the Monkey's management strategy cannot produce becomes available: genuine movement. The state shifts, because it is being met rather than managed.

Eugene Gendlin, the philosopher and psychotherapist who developed the Focusing technique, called this the felt sense – the bodily sense of a situation before it has been put into words. His decades of research into what makes therapy effective found that the patients who improved most were those who could attend to this pre-verbal bodily sense rather than immediately translating it into the Monkey's categories. The felt sense is the territory. The label is the map. Un-Naming is the practice of finding your way back to the territory – not to abandon the map, but to know the difference.

The Move That Changes Everything

In the Sōtō tradition of Zen Buddhism, there is an instruction that sounds, on first encounter, absurdly simple. When you are sitting in zazen and a thought or emotion arises, you do not attempt to suppress it, analyse it, or follow it. You simply note it: thinking. And return to the breath. Not to achieve a blank mind. To notice the arising of a mental event and to refuse, with great gentleness, to enter the narrative it is offering. Thinking. Return. Thinking. Return.

This instruction encodes one of the most practically consequential cognitive moves I know – a move that closes the gap between intellectually understanding the Naming Trap and the moment-by-moment lived practice of escaping it. And it has an analogue in everyday emotional life that does not require formal Zen training.

The move is this: from statement to sensation. Consider the statement I am angry. An autonomic state arises – a shift in arousal, a change in blood flow, a constellation of physiological events. Before any of this has been consciously encountered, the Monkey has named it, categorised it, incorporated it into identity, and drafted the beginning of a narrative. The 'I' is in place. The 'am' has promoted a transient physiological event into a stable property of the self. And 'angry' has recruited the entire semantic network associated with anger — its history, its justifications, its appropriate targets, its expected duration. All of this happens faster than conscious awareness. By the time you know you are angry, the Monkey has already built the room you are standing in.

The Un-Naming move is to interrupt this sequence at the level of physical sensation rather than at the level of the concept. Not I am angry but: there is heat in the chest. There is a contraction across the upper trapezius. The jaw has closed tightly. The breath has shortened and is sitting high in the sternum. The hands want to close. These are not translations of anger into poetic language. They are the encounter with what is actually present before anger has been assembled as a concept. They are the territory. I am angry is the map.

The Un-Naming move – practised consistently over time – introduces a gap into the self-confirming loop. Not by replacing 'I am angry' with 'I am calm' (which is merely one Monkey story replacing another), but by attending, with genuine curiosity, to what is physically present before the label is applied. The heat. The tightening. The breath. These are real. They are specific. They are present right now. And crucially – they are not stable. The heat is already changing as you attend to it. The tightening shifts as the breath lengthens. The territory, encountered directly, turns out to be dynamic, responsive, and considerably less fixed than the map insisted.

PRACTICE: *The Un-Naming Practice – Three Stages*

STAGE 1 – SENSATION (5 *minutes*):

Begin with the breathing practice. Then bring attention to any physical sensation.

When the label arrives, acknowledge it and set it gently aside. Ask instead: what is the raw quality of what is here? Pressure, heat, vibration, pulse, stillness? Stay with the actual sensation for as long as you can before the Monkey re-labels it. When it re-labels, set the label aside again. Return. This is the practice.

STAGE 2 – EMOTION (5 *minutes*):

Bring attention to your emotional state right now. Let the label come. Then ask: where in the body is this? Follow it as a sensation rather than a concept. Notice whether the state shifts when it is met directly rather than managed through its label.

STAGE 3 – OBSERVER (5 *minutes*):

Ask, gently: who is noticing all of this? Do not answer in words. Simply rest in the question itself, and notice what is there before the Monkey supplies an answer.

A necessary caution belongs here. If you are living with severe trauma or a trauma-related disorder, this approach may still be helpful, but it should be practised in coordination with a qualified healthcare provider or trauma-informed therapist. The point is not to force your way through activation. The point is to create enough safety that the system can begin to loosen without being overwhelmed.

Used in daily life, this protocol of proprioception, breathing, and Un-Naming can be remarkably practical. If I notice a headache beginning to gather, I will often use part of a lunch break for a short round of practice – a few minutes of slow breathing, several repetitions of the Un-Naming move, sometimes accompanied by gentle qigong. Quite often the headache settles before it fully develops. This is not a promise. It is a description of how quickly the organism can sometimes change direction when the story is dropped and the body is given a more accurate signal.

The Proprioception of Enlightenment

Proprioception-as-enlightenment is a description of what the contemplative traditions' most precise accounts of transformation actually point toward — and it connects directly to the body-based practices in this book.

Proprioception is the body's ongoing, pre-conscious awareness of its own position in space. The mechanoreceptors in the joints, the Golgi tendon organs, the muscle spindles, the vestibular system — these are continuously reporting the organism's configuration to the nervous system, below the level of conscious attention. What you are consciously aware of, in ordinary waking life, is the Monkey's summary of this information: a simplified, functional representation accurate enough for navigation and radically less detailed than the full proprioceptive picture.

What I mean by proprioception-as-enlightenment is this: the contemplative traditions' accounts of the awakened state — the state after the Monkey's habitual narration has been, at least temporarily, quieted — consistently describe an experience of extraordinary precision about physical reality. Not the Monkey's simplified summary but the territory itself, in its actual density of sensation and information. The meditator in deep practice is not floating in a pleasant vagueness. They are encountering the body's actual proprioceptive reality with an attention that the Monkey's compulsive narrating had been obscuring. The felt sense of the body's aliveness – the specific quality of sensation in each region, the continuous micro-adjustments of balance and breath and circulation – becomes available in a richness that ordinary awareness does not access.

This is, I believe, what the Zen instruction 'thinking, return' is actually training. Not the suppression of thought but the development of a capacity to return from thought to sensation – to the actual proprioceptive and interoceptive reality of the body in this moment – with sufficient speed and reliability that the interval between thought-arising and return-to-sensation becomes shorter and shorter. In Zen this is sometimes called shikantaza – just sitting.

Not sitting with a goal, not sitting to produce a state. Just sitting, with the full proprioceptive attention of the organism fully present with what is actually here. The instruction is deceptively simple. What it requires, developed over years of sustained practice, is a degree of somatic attention that most people have never been asked to cultivate. We are trained, from early childhood, to attend to content – to ideas, objects, narratives. We are almost never trained to attend to the medium: the body that is having the experience, the proprioceptive field in which all content arises.

The Un-Naming Practice, in this frame, is not merely a technique for emotional regulation – though it is that too. It is an introduction to proprioceptive attention. A way of beginning to develop the capacity – and it is a capacity, requiring consistent use to strengthen – of returning to the body's actual present-moment reality rather than to the Monkey's story about it.

Unlearning as a Positive Practice

The Daodejing's formulation in Chapter 48 is by now familiar: in pursuit of the Dao, every day something is dropped. What is subtracted are Friston's priors – the thickened certainties that the nervous system has confused with reality.

The neuroscientific analogue is not comforting to the Monkey. Learning – the formation of new long-term potentiation, the reinforcement of synaptic pathways – requires effort, repetition, and the expenditure of metabolic resources. Unlearning – the revision of deeply held predictive models – requires something the brain does not do easily or naturally:

sustained prediction error. The repeated, unignorable encounter with evidence that the existing model is wrong.

This is why the contemplative traditions' practices are so demanding, and why the simple instruction 'return to the breath' contains such difficulty. The Monkey's model – its story about who you are, what the world is, what is about to happen – is reinforced by decades of experience. Every confirmed prediction strengthens the model. The practice of returning – again and again and again – to the actual sensation of the breath, rather than to the Monkey's narrative about the breath or the meditation or the progress being made, is a practice of generating the prediction error that unlearning requires. The Monkey predicts: now I will plan what I need to do later. Return. The Monkey predicts: now I will evaluate how well I am meditating. Return. Each return is a small, accurate moment of the model being wrong. Each return is unlearning applied at the grain of a single moment.

Over time – and this is the honest account of what the practice actually produces, rather than the idealised narrative – the model changes. Not dramatically, not permanently, not finally. But the Monkey's grip loosens, incrementally, in proportion to the accumulated prediction error. The intervals of genuine somatic presence become longer. The return from narrative to sensation becomes faster. The proprioceptive reality of the body becomes more available as a ground state. Not because you have achieved anything. Because you have, very gradually, learned to stop doing the thing that was preventing you from inhabiting it. This is what Sōtō Zen means by practice-enlightenment — shusha-itto, the unity of practice and realisation. Enlightenment is not a destination reached at the end of the practice. It is present, in miniature, in every genuine moment of return. The territory is not at the end of the path. It is in every step in which you stop following the map.

What the body knew:

The label is not the enemy. The label is the Monkey's gift — the tool that makes navigation possible. But the label is not the thing. Between the sensation and the name, there is a moment of pure encounter that the practice of Un-Naming is designed to lengthen. In that moment, the body is already practising what the mind is still learning to allow.

Releasing the Story from the Tissue

"The hard and stiff belong to death. The soft and yielding belong to life"

– Daodejing, Chapter 76

Self-Myofascial Work as Narrative Practice

If the stories are stored in the tissue, the tissue can be asked – with patience, with presence, with the right quality of sustained attention – to release them. Not by telling a different story. By attending to what the tissue is actually holding, before the story has been applied. This chapter is the most direct available translation of everything Part II established: the body keeps its records, and the body can be invited to release them.

This chapter is about working directly with that stored material. Not through clinical intervention – that requires a trained practitioner's hands and years of palpatory sensitivity – but through what you can reach from the inside, with patience, with presence, and with the right quality of attention.

Let me be clear about what this is not before we begin. This is not wellness maintenance. This is not self-care in the sense the wellness industry means it — a reward for the week's effort. When you apply sustained pressure to a restricted area of your own fascia and hold the breath steady through the discomfort and feel the tissue slowly release, you are interrupting a story that has been running in your body, sometimes for years. You are giving the Monkey's somatic correlate a chance to update. That requires the same quality of direct, patient, non-narrating attention that the preceding chapters have been training. The breath is the foundation. Un-Naming is the companion. What follows is the territory they open into.

The One Principle That Changes Everything

Most people's instinct about releasing tension is to push harder. To override the restriction with sufficient intensity. This is how we approach most physical problems. The fascia does not respond to this. Or rather, it responds briefly — the tissue yields to acute force and then returns, usually within hours, to exactly its previous state. Because the force reached the muscle, not the fascia. And it did not reach the story.

Fascia responds to low load applied over a long duration. This is its viscoelastic nature. Under sustained, gentle pressure, the ground substance – the hydrated gel that fills the spaces between the collagen fibres – gradually shifts its viscosity. It becomes more fluid. The fibres can move relative to each other. The restriction releases. And crucially, this release happens slowly enough that the nervous system can register it – can update its predictive model of what this area is doing, can revise the chronic prediction of tension and threat that has been maintaining the pattern.

Find the barrier: the first edge of resistance, well before pain. Stop there. Breathe into it with the LSD rhythm. Hold for a minimum of ninety seconds, and preferably considerably longer. Feel for the gradual softening – not a dramatic pop or snap, but a slow, spreading warmth, a sense of the tissue yielding not to force but to time. Then wait a little longer. The release continues after you think it has finished.

I saw this demonstrated clearly in a patient I worked with in the early years of my Ho Chi Minh City practice — a Vietnamese woman in her late fifties with chronic restriction through the anterior hip and lower thorax that had been present for so long she had stopped experiencing it as restriction and simply experienced it as herself. We had worked together for several sessions with modest results. Then, at the fourth session, she arrived having spent a week using the diaphragm and psoas release positions at home each morning for fifteen minutes. The tissue under my hands that day was different — not dramatically, but unmistakably. Something had begun to change its mind. She had not achieved this through force. She had stayed at the first edge of resistance, consistently enough and long enough, that the fascial ground substance had begun to shift. The improvement in that session built on work the tissue had already started doing for itself. This is what the practices in this chapter are designed to support: not the dramatic release of the treatment table, but the slow, daily undoing that the tissue is capable of when it is met with patience rather than effort.

Where the Stories Live

Clinical work has given me a strong sense of where stories tend to concentrate. I offer what follows not as a rigid system but as a map — remembering always that the map is not the territory, and that your own body's record is more accurate than any generalisation I can provide.

In my clinical experience, the diaphragm often becomes part of the physical pattern associated with sustained stress — the chronic bracing against a world that feels threatening, the breath held at half-capacity for years without the Monkey noticing. When the diaphragm is restricted, breathing is shallow, the vagus nerve is under-stimulated, and the Monkey's stress narrative has a permanent physiological anchor. The organism is perpetually in a state of mild preparation. Releasing the diaphragm is one of the most direct routes to parasympathetic activation available outside of clinical treatment. Lie on your back, knees bent, feet flat. Place the fingertips gently beneath the lower ribs on both sides. On the exhale, allow the fingertips to follow the ribs inward and upward very slightly as the diaphragm ascends. Maintain that gentle contact through the next inhale, feeling the ribs expand against your fingers. Stay for several breath cycles. You are not stretching anything. You are reminding the tissue that movement is available here.

In my clinical experience, the psoas often becomes part of the physical pattern associated with unresolved threat – the sustained vigilance of a nervous system that has never been given clear permission to stand down. The chronic fight-or-flight that was activated but never completed. The psoas is the only muscle that connects the spine directly to the leg. When it is chronically shortened – in almost everyone who sits for extended periods, and in many people who have lived through sustained stress or trauma – it pulls the lumbar spine forward, compresses the sacrum, restricts the breath, and maintains a biological posture that the Monkey narrates as: something is wrong. Something requires vigilance. I must stay ready. A sustained lunge position reaches the psoas where most stretches cannot. Rear knee on the floor, front shin vertical, torso upright. Hold for three to five minutes – not thirty seconds, but long enough for the viscoelastic creep to begin. Breathe slowly and completely into the front of the rear hip. Do not lean into the stretch. Simply arrive at the barrier and remain there.

In my clinical experience, the upper trapezius and posterior neck often become part of the physical pattern associated with carrying – with responsibility, with the Monkey's perpetual agenda, with the weight of everything that must be managed. The shoulders that never fully descend. For self-myofascial release, I often suggest using tools such as tennis balls, lacrosse balls, fascia rollers, or any other tool your body responds well to. Place a lacrosse ball or tennis ball between the upper trapezius and the wall. Apply body weight gently by leaning back into it. Find a point of density and stop. Do not roll. Rolling tells the nervous system that the pressure is temporary and passing; the tissue simply waits for it to move on. Anchoring – finding the restriction, arriving, and staying – is what creates the conditions for the tissue to change. Hold for sixty to ninety seconds per point. Breathe. When the density softens, move to the adjacent area.

In my clinical experience, the soles of the feet often carry a pattern related to contact with the ground – or, more precisely, to its absence. The plantar fascia is the beginning of the Superficial Back Line, the fascial continuity that runs from the soles of the feet up the back of the legs, along the spine, and over the skull to the forehead. What is held in the feet is not local. It ripples upward through the entire posterior chain. A tennis ball is the right tool: firm enough to reach the plantar fascia, yielding enough not to overwhelm it. Stand on it barefoot, with enough body weight to feel the pressure without pain. Move from point to point – pausing wherever the tissue feels dense, staying for thirty to sixty seconds before advancing. Cross the arch. Reach the ball of the foot. What you will likely notice, when you first do this attentively, is how much information the soles contain. Areas of density you were not aware of. Asymmetries between left and right. You are not just releasing plantar fascia. You are restoring the body's primary interface with the earth it stands on.

A Note on What Follows Significant Release

A meaningful fascial release can be accompanied by a sudden shift in emotional state that seems entirely disproportionate to what you were doing physically. Tears arriving from nowhere. A wave of something that is not quite fear and not quite sadness but needs to move through. A sudden quality of lightness where there had been nothing but familiar weight. This is not unusual. In the EMFT model, this is release rather than accumulation: tissue that had been holding a pattern is letting it go. Allow it to move. The breath is the guide: keep it slow, steady, and nasal even as the emotion rises. It will pass. Something more spacious arrives after.

The Monkey, at this point, will want a sequence. A clear protocol. A numbered list of exactly what to do and in what order. I understand this. But a fixed protocol tells the nervous system what is going to happen next, which means the nervous system is already predicting and bracing rather than listening. Begin instead with a few minutes of LSD breathing – Light, Slow, Deep, the foundation practice from Chapter 11 – enough to establish the parasympathetic baseline that the tissue needs in order to release at all. Then ask: where is the Monkey holding on today? You will know. The body has been reporting this continuously; you have simply been filtering the signal. Bring the tool to that area. Arrive. Stay. Breathe. Wait for the release, and then wait a little longer. Move when the tissue invites movement, not when the clock says it is time.

The same protocol can also accompany professional treatment. Massage, myofascial release, guided stretching, and related hands-on approaches often become more effective when the body is first brought into a quieter state through slow nasal breathing and the proprioceptive, Un-Naming attention developed in the preceding chapters. In my experience, dropping the story while the physical work is being done allows the tissue and the narrative to update together. They are, as this book has argued throughout, one process perceived from two angles.

What the body knew:

In this model, the body does not store stories as abstractions. It stores them as physical patterns – fascial restrictions, altered tension, compressed spaces where fluid has ceased to move freely. Releasing those patterns is not merely physical maintenance. It is the practice of intellectual honesty applied to the tissue. It is asking the body: what are you actually holding here? And then – with patience, with presence, without forcing — allowing the honest answer to emerge.

Entering the Flow

"In the pursuit of learning, one accumulates daily. In the pursuit of the way, one diminishes daily. Diminishing and again diminishing, until one arrives at non-action. Through non-action, nothing is left undone."

— Daodejing, Chapter 48

The Practice of Boundlessness

Everything in this book has been preparation for what this chapter cannot give you.

The state that Newberg documented — parietal quieting, DMN deactivation, the dissolution of the self-other boundary — cannot be directly produced by technique. This is not because it is supernatural or reserved for the spiritually advanced. It is because the state, by definition, involves the temporary suspension of the very apparatus that is trying to produce it. The Monkey cannot engineer the Monkey's own silence.

The technique cannot dissolve the technician. What practice can do is create the conditions under which the silence becomes more available. To use the river as the Daodejing uses it: the river does not force its way to the sea. It follows the path of least resistance, yielding to what is, and by yielding, it arrives. Practice is not forcing the arrival. It is removing the obstacles to the natural flow.

Sitting With the Gap

I have been meditating seriously for well over a decade — long before the summer of 2022, when, over several weeks of unusually deep practice, the boundary between self and surroundings thinned to the point of briefly disappearing altogether — with increasing depth and frequency as the years have passed. What I have actually found in that practice is different in several respects from what the popular accounts of meditation suggest, and I want to share what is real rather than what is reassuring.

The first thing I found was that the Monkey is far louder in the silence than it is in the noise of daily life. The moment I sat and closed my eyes, the commentary intensified. Plans, memories, self-assessments, sudden urgent tasks – the Monkey, deprived of external stimulation to narrate, turned inward with considerable energy. This is normal. It is what the DMN does when freed from external task-engagement. It is not a sign of failure or an unsuitable mind. It is the beginning.

The second thing I found was that the instruction to 'clear the mind' is both wrong and, for most beginners, counterproductive. The mind does not clear. The Monkey does not stop. The practice is not the production of silence but the development of a particular relationship to the noise – the ability to observe the commentary without being carried by it. To notice the thought without adding the next thought to it.

The third thing – arriving more slowly, after months of regular practice – was that the commentary began to develop gaps. Not long ones at first. A second or two of genuine quiet between the Monkey's sentences. But those gaps had a quality that was unmistakable: a sense of presence, of aliveness, of direct contact with the present moment that the narrative had been obscuring. And in those gaps, sometimes – not always, not reliably, but often enough to reorient everything – something larger became briefly available. The boundlessness. The felt sense of the self-other boundary becoming permeable. What I wrote in my journal as feeling more real than reality.

PRACTICE: *The Gap Practice*

Sit comfortably, spine upright but not rigid. Eyes closed or softly downcast. Establish the LSD breath: Light, Slow, Deep, through the nose. Let the breath settle for two to three minutes before anything else.

Bring attention to the breath itself – not as a technique to be performed, but as a living event happening in the body. The physical sensation of air moving. The rise and fall of the belly. The slight pause between the exhale and the next inhale.

When thoughts arise — and they will — do not fight them. Do not follow them into their content. Simply note: thinking. And return to the breath. Not with frustration. With the same patient curiosity you would bring to a physical sensation in the Un-Naming practice.

As the session deepens, the gaps between thoughts will lengthen. When a gap arrives, do not name it or reach toward it. Simply rest in it, for as long as it lasts. The gap will close. The Monkey will return. This is not failure. Return to the breath. The next gap will come.

Begin with 10 to 20 minutes daily. Over weeks and months, extend to 45 or 60 minutes if possible. Some sessions will be almost entirely Monkey. This is not wasted time. The act of returning — of sitting with the noise without being swept away by it — is itself the practice.

Movement as an Entry Point

Not everyone finds stillness the easiest gateway. For some bodies – particularly those carrying significant chronic tension, or those whose Monkey is particularly activated by the absence of external stimulus – movement is the more accessible entry point. Qigong, introduced earlier in this book, is not exercise in the conventional sense; its purpose is to cultivate what practitioners call Qi, which I understand, in the framework of this book, as the free and unobstructed flow of biological process through the liquid matrix of the fascial web. The core instruction of Qigong is simple enough to state and demanding enough to practise: every movement is coordinated with the breath, every breath is slow and nasal, and the quality of attention is the same Un-Naming quality we have been cultivating – present, curious, non-evaluative. The movement is not performed. It is inhabited.

When movement is inhabited in this way – when the attention is fully in the body, following the sensation rather than narrating it – something begins to happen that those who have experienced it recognise immediately. The Monkey quiets. Not because it has been suppressed but because the body's attention is so full that the narrative circuits do not have their usual purchase. This is the flow state Csikszentmihalyi describes – self-consciousness withdrawing, the action and the actor becoming, briefly, one. Wu Wei made embodied: the living experience of an organism moving in accord with its own nature, without the friction of a Monkey simultaneously trying to manage, evaluate, and narrate the movement. The principle can be applied to walking – slow, conscious walking in which each step is felt rather than thought. To swimming. To dancing. To any form of movement you know well enough that the technique requires no conscious effort, and that you are willing to inhabit rather than perform. The question to ask of any movement practice: am I doing this, or is it happening? The answer, when you are genuinely in the flow, is always both. You become the happening. And the boundary between the two has temporarily dissolved.

Three Further Practices

Beyond the gap practice and the qigong principle, three practices have proven particularly valuable in my own experience and in my work with patients. I offer them not as a sequence but as a toolkit – to be explored in whatever order the body finds most open.

1. *The Boundless Body Scan*

Most body scan practices move attention systematically through the body region by region, noting sensations as they go. This is a valuable starting point. But it has a structural limitation: it reinforces the Monkey's map of the body as a collection of discrete parts. The Boundless Body Scan is different in structure and intention. Rather than moving through the body, it begins with the widest possible field of somatic attention and asks: what is the body as a whole doing right now? Not what is each part doing, but what is the global state of the organism in this moment?

The aim is to encounter the fascial web as it actually is – continuous, uninterrupted, global – rather than as the anatomical map presents it.

Begin with the breath established, nasal, slow, and diaphragmatic. Then expand the field of attention outward from the breath until it is resting, as lightly as possible, on the entire organism simultaneously. Not scanning from foot to head. Simply being present to the whole. Notice what presents itself without directing attention toward it. This is the proprioceptive equivalent of peripheral vision – not focusing, but receiving. If the Monkey begins to parse the experience into parts, gently widen the attention back to the whole. Not denying the particular sensation, but holding it within the larger field rather than isolating it.

What often happens, particularly as the practice deepens over weeks and months, is that the edge of the body becomes less fixed. Not that the physical boundary disappears. But the quality of attention changes. The skin, encountered this way, stops being a wall and becomes more like a membrane – a region of particularly dense sensation within a larger field that extends into the space around the body. This is not a mystical claim. It is the natural consequence of attending to the fascial web's actual sensory reality, which includes a considerable density of mechanoreceptors in the skin and subcutaneous fascia – described by some researchers as among the richest sensory tissues in the body – that, under ordinary conditions, feed into the Monkey's simplified body image rather than being encountered directly. A caveat: this practice is not suitable as a starting point for people carrying unresolved trauma, or for those whose autonomic state is significantly dysregulated. If it produces discomfort or anxiety rather than spaciousness, return to the 5:5 breathing practice and build a longer foundation there before returning here.

2. *The Practice of Not-Knowing*

This is the simplest practice in the book, and the hardest. It has no technique. It has only a quality of orientation.

Sit comfortably. Breathe in the LSD pattern. Allow the eyes to close. And then – rather than directing attention anywhere, rather than scanning or observing or returning from thought – simply rest in the question: what is actually happening right now? Not as a cognitive inquiry. Not with the intention of formulating an answer. As a genuinely open orientation to present-moment reality, in which the honest answer – I do not know what is happening right now; I know the Monkey's story about it, but not the thing itself – is held without anxiety, without urgency, and without the Monkey's compulsive need to resolve it into a completed account.

This is what the Daodejing means by wu zhi – not-knowing. Not ignorance. Not the absence of information. The active, chosen orientation of the practised mind toward the territory, rather than toward its own map. The sage, in Chapter 71, knows without knowing. The knowledge that precedes and underlies the Monkey's categories. The direct encounter with what is, before the question of what to call it.

The Monkey will arrive almost immediately with an answer. Set it gently aside. Return to the open question. Not-knowing is not produced by effort. It is what is present when the effort to know is, for this moment, released. Spend five minutes here, initially. Return to the breath if the practice produces disorientation. Over time, the capacity to rest in genuine not-knowing develops its own stability. The open question becomes a ground rather than an absence. The uncarved block: not nothing, but the condition of possibility for everything.

3. *Entering Flow Through Contact*

The experiences of that summer — the dissolution of the self-other boundary, the quality of boundlessness that arose in deep meditative states — did not occur primarily in formal sitting practice. They occurred in moments of deep contact: with patients on the treatment table, with the particular quality of attention that sustained clinical work produces, with the tissue speaking back through the hands.

The dominant image of contemplative practice in the Western secular context is the solitary meditator. And there is something important and irreplaceable in the solitary practice. But the nervous system was not built for solitude. It was built for resonance. The ventral vagal state – the physiological substrate of genuine presence and openness – was evolved in the context of social engagement. It is most naturally activated in the presence of other regulated, open, present nervous systems. The co-regulation that Porges describes is not a supplement to the primary practice of internal regulation. For many people, it is the more natural entry point.

Contact, in the sense I mean here, is not merely physical. It is the quality of attention that occurs when two nervous systems are genuinely present to each other – when the Monkey's normal agenda of self-presentation, management, and strategic interpretation is sufficiently relaxed that something more direct becomes possible. You have experienced this. The conversation in which time disappeared.

The activity shared with another person in which you lost track of who was doing what. The moment of genuine recognition – of being seen and seeing – that is qualitatively different from ordinary social exchange. These are moments of ventral vagal co-regulation, of the self-other boundary becoming temporarily more permeable. They are, in neurological terms, the social version of the meditative dissolution.

The practice of entering flow through contact is not a technique. It is an orientation: the willingness to arrive in the presence of another person – or in the engagement with a task, or in the encounter with a piece of music or a landscape – with the Un-Naming quality of attention the preceding chapters have been building. Without an agenda. Without the Monkey's pre-written account of what is about to happen. Meeting what is actually there rather than the story you have already drafted about it. This is what the Daodejing calls wu wei applied to relation: effortless action arising from genuine presence rather than strategic intention. It cannot be practised as a technique, because the moment you are applying a technique, the technique is what is present, not the contact. It arises, when it arises, as the natural consequence of sufficient Un-Naming. The territory, encountered honestly enough, turns out to be full of other territories. The web, seen clearly, is full of other weavings.

The Bridge Toward Silence

I want to be careful, at the end of this chapter, about what I am claiming for these practices. I have spent this entire book resisting the Monkey's preference for a closed and satisfying conclusion – resisting the temptation to offer the experience of resolution where resolution is not actually available. I am not going to violate that commitment now, with the finish line in sight.

The practices work. I have watched them work in my own life and in the lives of the patients who have committed to them. Not dramatically, not uniformly, not for everyone, and not in the way the Monkey would prefer – as a linear, predictable progression toward a clearly defined destination. They work the way water works on stone: slowly, continuously, following the path of least resistance, asking nothing except time and repetition. The stone does not experience a dramatic moment of dissolution. It simply, one day, is shaped differently than it was.

What the practices produce, for most people and over most of the time, is not enlightenment. It is something more modest and more durable: a gradual increase in the proportion of time spent in the territory rather than the map. More moments of genuine somatic presence. A slightly faster return from the Monkey's narrative to the breath, the sensation, the unmediated encounter with what is actually here. A loosening of the stories that have been maintained, at some cost, by the tissue and the nervous system together. A growing familiarity with the quality of silence that exists between the Monkey's sentences – and a growing trust that the silence is not empty.

Those experiences deserve a brief return. The experience of boundlessness, when it comes, does not feel like a neurological event. It feels like contact with something that was always there – something the ordinary sense of a separate self had been obscuring. Not a new discovery but a recognition. A returning to something that was, in some sense, always already home. Is this the Dao? Is it the organism briefly perceiving its own fundamental nature? Is it the hard problem becoming briefly transparent – the felt sense of existence before the Monkey builds a story around it? I do not know. I am genuinely uncertain. And I have come to believe that the uncertainty itself – held without panic, without the urgent need for a story to fill it – is part of the practice.

I do not know what lies in that silence. I have experienced it. I have found it, consistently and without exception, to be something rather than nothing – a quality of presence, of aliveness, of what I can only call love in its most literal and least sentimental sense. But I cannot tell you what it is. Every attempt to name it would be the Monkey reasserting itself, and the naming would replace the thing. What I can tell you is that it is always there. It was there before you began this book and it will be there after you set it down. The practices are not producing it. They are removing what has been obscuring it. The territory is not a destination. It is where you already are, when the map is, for once, set aside.

What the body knew:

The state that the practices point toward is not a reward for sufficient effort. It is what is already present when the Monkey's effort ceases. The practices do not produce the silence. They remove, gradually and honestly, the habits that prevent the silence from being noticed. The river does not work to reach the sea. It simply flows, and the sea is already at the end of every flow.

PART FOUR

Beyond the Map

Uncertainty, humility, and what remains when the map is set aside

Afterword

Embracing the Fascial Web: A Journey of Connection and Potential

This book has aimed to provide not just information, but a new lens through which to view the human body. To move beyond the outdated model of isolated muscles and bones, and to embrace the concept of a truly interconnected web – a living matrix that responds to our every thought, movement, and experience.

Steve's life, much like the fascial web he studies, is a continuous journey of exploration, a quest to find harmony and meaning in the ever-changing currents of existence. He invites you, the reader, to join him on this path, to contemplate the timeless wisdom found within these pages, and to discover your own way in the ever-flowing river of wellness.

As you journeyed through these pages, you may have noticed the occasional resonance with ancient wisdom – traces of the Daodejing, whose acceptance of natural order, wisdom found in stillness, and surrender to what cannot be controlled have become a guiding principle in my own life and practice. Its imagery of water – yielding, yet wearing down what is hard – offers a fitting metaphor for fascia itself, and for the letting go that fascia-puncture, at its best, requires. This same humility applies to the knowledge in this book: I hold it as adaptable, subject to revision, and secondary to what your own hands and your own body's evidence will teach you.

The Daodejing has been such steady company on this path that I did not want to leave it as a handful of scattered lines between chapters. What follows the reading list, in the appendix, is one of my own renderings of Laozi's eighty-one chapters – the version I call The Unnamed River. It stands on its own there, not as illustration for anything in the preceding pages, but simply as the text that has quietly shaped how I think and work. Read it, or don't; either way, it will still be here.

Since the first edition, the investigation has gone further. Writing The Storytelling Monkey and the Web of Life forced me to confront what I had been observing in clinical work for years: that the fascial web is not merely a structural system. It is the primary somatic site of the stories the brain tells about who we are. The Default Mode Network generates the narrative. The predictive hierarchy maintains it. And the fascia — living, innervated, mechanically responsive — is where that narrative takes up physical residence. Releasing the tissue and releasing the story are not two different interventions. They are two names for the same act, entered from different ends of the same reality. The body knew this before the words arrived. It always does.

A Request in Closing

If this book has touched something in you – raised a question, shifted a thought – I would be very glad if you took a moment to leave a short review on the website of the retailer where you purchased it. Such feedback is not only encouraging for an independent author – it helps the book reach the people it was written for. And if you know someone in your circle who engages with questions of consciousness, embodiment, or the great questions of life: a personal recommendation is the most sincere thing a book can wish for. The web of life is also woven between people who pass each other something worth reading. Thank you sincerely.

About the Author

Steve Brandl – Bridging Worlds for a Deeper Understanding of Fascia

Born in the green heart of Thuringia, Germany, Steve Brandl's professional journey has been a testament to bridging seemingly disparate worlds in the pursuit of holistic health. His foundational education in healthcare, culminating in his work in physical therapy and the implementation of various medical massage therapies, provided him with a profound appreciation for the intricate mechanics of the human body through the lens of modern Western science. This initial exploration, however, ignited a deeper curiosity, drawing him towards the profound wisdom inherent in ancient healing traditions.

Driven by this thirst for comprehensive understanding, Steve immersed himself in the study of acupuncture and traditional medicine, eventually becoming a certified health practitioner – Heilpraktiker. This profound engagement with Eastern philosophies and healing practices, particularly his decade-long immersion in Vietnam as a practising acupuncturist, has shaped his unique approach. In his daily clinical work, Steve masterfully weaves together the insights of cutting-edge fascia research with the timeless principles of acupuncture and traditional medicine. This unique integration allows him to view the body not just as a collection of parts, but as an interconnected fascial web, seeking to unlock its innate capacity for healing and balance.

Steve is the author of the From Nothing to Infinity series of Daodejing translations and of The Storytelling Monkey and the Web of Life (2026), which explores the neuroscience of the self, the body as the primary site of stored narrative, and the territory where science meets the boundary it cannot cross.

Steve's approach is deeply informed by his core belief in the interconnectedness of all things – a principle that extends beyond the physical realm into the philosophical inquiries that resonate with him. The great mysteries of being, the nature of reality, and the essence of truth have long occupied his thoughts, forming the bedrock for his profound contemplations on the body's subtle energies and structural integrity.

He is a devoted husband and loving father, finding harmony and inspiration in the rhythms of family life, which mirror the delicate balance he seeks to understand in the wider universe and within the human body.

In moments of respite, Steve finds solace and renewal in the gentle movements of Qigong, the rhythmic cadence of bicycle rides through the Vietnamese landscape, and the quiet communion with the natural world. These grounding practices serve as constant reminders of the subtle dance between stillness and movement, the yin and yang that underpin all of existence, and which are so beautifully reflected in the dynamic physiology of fascia.

A note on sources: the opening chapter, "The Making of a Fascia-Puncturist," is adapted from Chapter 9 of The Storytelling Monkey: Where Neuroscience ends and Wisdom begins (2026). The Investigation, in Part II, is adapted from Part I of The Uncarved Block: An Encounter with Laozi & Zhuangzi. The practice chapters in Part III are adapted from Part III of The Storytelling Monkey. The Unnamed River, in the appendix, is reproduced in full from the author's own rendering of the Daodejing of the same name.

The Unnamed River

Laozi's Daodejing, rendered by Steve Brandl

Eighty-one chapters, offered here in full and in their own right — not as illustration for anything in the preceding pages, but as a text that stands on its own.

Chapter 1

What can be explained is not the whole Way.

What can be named is not the whole source.

Before we divide life into words,

there is a deeper reality.

Once we name things,

we begin to manage and compare them.

Both the nameless and the named

belong to one reality.

One shows its depth.

The other shows its forms.

To live well, look through appearances

back to the source.

Chapter 2

The moment we praise one thing as beautiful,

we create the idea of ugliness.

The moment we praise one thing as good,

we create the idea of its opposite.

Life moves by contrast.

Being and non-being define each other.

Difficult and easy depend on each other.

The wise person does not force

a fixed identity onto things.

They do the work that needs doing.

Then they let it stand on its own.

Chapter 3

Do not excite envy by glorifying status.

Do not stir greed by displaying rare possessions.

Do not confuse people by feeding endless desire.

Good leadership calms the mind and simplifies life.

It gives people enough.

It weakens vanity and strengthens what is essential.

When ambition is not constantly inflamed,

people find their balance.

When life is not overmanaged,

it can settle into order.

Chapter 4

The Way is like an empty vessel.

Because it is empty, it can always be used.

Because it is never full of itself,

it is never exhausted.

It softens sharpness.

It untangles knots.

It lowers glare.

It joins what has been separated.

It is subtle, hidden, and yet the source

of what endures.

Chapter 5

Nature is not sentimental.

It does not reward one thing

and punish another to satisfy human preference.

It allows all things to follow their course.

The wise person learns from this.

They do not cling to private bias.

They make room for what is.

The space within a bellows looks empty,

yet it gives power.

The quieter the center,

the more life can move through it.

Chapter 6

The deep source never runs dry.

It is like a hidden valley

that keeps giving birth.

It is quiet, receptive, and inexhaustible.

What is most fruitful

is often what is least conspicuous.

Stay close to that hidden source.

Do not assume that power must look dramatic.

Much of life is sustained by what remains unseen.

Chapter 7

Heaven and earth endure

because they do not live for themselves.

The wise person becomes trustworthy

for the same reason.

By not putting themselves first,

they are not easily threatened.

By not guarding the self so tightly,

they become fully present.

What is done without self-importance lasts longer.

What is given without grasping returns in due time.

Chapter 8

The highest goodness is like water.

Water benefits everything without competing.

It goes to the low places others avoid.

That is why it resembles the Way.

In daily life, choose what is solid and simple.

In thought, stay clear.

In relationship, stay sincere.

In action, act at the right moment

rather than with force.

Chapter 9

Better to stop before excess becomes collapse.

A cup filled to the rim cannot be carried far.

A blade kept too sharp will not last.

A house crowded with gold invites fear.

Success followed by self-display leads to loss.

Do your work well.

Then step back.

This is how completion stays whole.

Chapter 10

Can you hold body and mind

together without strain.

Can you stay flexible

without losing integrity.

Can you keep your inner vision clear

without forcing certainty.

Can you care for people

without controlling them.

Can you act without possession.

Can you guide without domination.

To create, to nurture, to serve,

and not to claim ownership:

this is deep virtue.

Chapter 11

Thirty spokes meet at the hub,

but the usefulness of the wheel

is in the empty center.

Clay becomes a cup,

but the usefulness of the cup

is in the hollow space.

Walls make a room,

but the usefulness of the room

is in what is open.

Form matters.

Emptiness makes form usable.

Chapter 12

Too much stimulation makes perception dull.

Too much noise makes listening weak.

Too much craving unsettles the heart.

Too much chasing after novelty confuses judgment.

The wise person does not live from surface appetite.

They return to what nourishes life more deeply.

They do not feed every impulse.

They protect inner clarity.

Chapter 13

Favor and disgrace both disturb the mind

when identity depends on them.

Gain and loss both create anxiety

when the self is overprotected.

Why are we troubled.

Because we cling to an image of ourselves.

Care for your life,

but do not worship your image.

Then responsibility becomes natural

rather than fearful.

One who can care for life without vanity

can be trusted with greater things.

Chapter 14

Look for the Way

and you cannot see it as an object.

Listen for it and you cannot hear it as a sound.

Reach for it and you cannot seize it as a thing.

It cannot be reduced to the senses.

It is subtle, continuous, and prior to appearances.

Follow it back and you meet the source.

Follow it forward and you see its effects.

To live in the present,

stay connected to that continuity.

Chapter 15

The old masters were careful,

quiet, and hard to read.

Not because they were obscure,

but because they would not pretend

to know too much.

They were alert

like one crossing winter water.

Open like a valley.

Simple like uncarved wood.

Patient with what had not yet settled.

When muddy water is left alone, it clears.

When life is not rushed, the right shape appears.

Chapter 16

Reach for deep stillness.

Keep returning to inner quiet.

Then you can watch all things

rise and pass without panic.

Everything blooms.

Everything returns to its root.

Returning to the root is rest.

Rest reveals the pattern.

Seeing the pattern gives steadiness.

Without that steadiness,

action becomes reckless.

Chapter 17

The best leader is barely felt.

Next comes the one who is loved.

Then the one who is feared.

Then the one who is despised.

When trust is lacking, trust cannot grow.

The best leader speaks little.

They do the work.

Things are set in order.

And people say: we did it ourselves.

Chapter 18

When the great Way is forgotten,

moral slogans multiply.

When natural affection weakens,

dutiful performance is praised.

When family harmony is broken,

talk of obedience grows loud.

When a state is in confusion,

public virtue becomes a display.

Do not mistake noise for health.

When life is aligned,

goodness does not need advertisement.

Chapter 19

Drop cleverness and people benefit.

Drop rigid moral posturing

and people recover ordinary kindness.

Drop greed for profit and theft loses its lure.

These reforms sound simple,

but they must reach the heart.

Live plainly.

Value what is natural.

Reduce selfish calculation.

Return to what is genuine.

Chapter 20

Stop living by every social approval

and disapproval.

How great is the difference between yes and no

when the heart is unsettled.

Most people rush after occasions and appearances.

The wise person stays rooted.

Others seek excitement.

The wise person values nourishment.

Others shine outwardly.

The wise person remains close to the source.

Chapter 21

Deep virtue follows the Way

and not private preference.

The Way is elusive and hard to grasp,

yet within it are patterns,

possibilities, and life.

Its truth is not always obvious,

but it is reliable.

From ancient times until now,

it has never ceased.

Through it we can recognize

the origin of all things.

We know the source by the quality

of what it brings forth.

Chapter 22

What is bent can become straight.

What is hollow can be filled.

What is worn can be renewed.

What has little is not yet trapped by excess.

What has too much is often confused.

The wise person does not insist on self-display.

So they are seen clearly.

They do not justify themselves.

So they are trusted.

By not competing,

they cannot easily be defeated.

Chapter 23

Few words carry farther than many.

A whirlwind does not last all morning.

A storm does not last all day.

Nature does not force intensity

beyond its season.

Why should we.

One who lives in accord with the Way

becomes aligned with it.

One who lives by virtue

becomes strengthened by it.

One who lives by loss

becomes familiar with loss.

What we practice, we join.

Chapter 24

One who stands on tiptoe cannot stand steadily.

One who strides to show off does not walk well.

One who is obsessed with being seen is not clear.

One who praises themselves is not convincing.

One who clings to achievement

loses the freshness of action.

From the perspective of the Way,

these are like excess baggage.

They burden life rather than serve it.

Chapter 25

There is something formless yet complete,

present before heaven and earth took shape.

Quiet, empty, unforced, and unchanging,

it moves through everything and is never exhausted.

I do not know its proper name.

I call it the Way.

It is great because it flows.

It flows because it goes beyond itself.

It returns because what is true completes a circle.

Chapter 26

Weight is the root of lightness.

Stillness is the master of restlessness.

A person of depth carries calm within motion.

Therefore the wise do not lose their center

in the midst of activity.

Though there may be sights worth seeing,

they do not abandon what is essential

for what is exciting.

One who is ruled by agitation

loses command of self.

Chapter 27

A good traveler leaves no needless trace.

A good speaker does not need

to trap others in argument.

A good accountant works

without anxiety over tally.

A good door needs no lock

if nothing invites theft.

A good bond needs no cord

if trust is real.

The wise person does not reject people.

They know how to use each situation.

This is called following the hidden

intelligence of life.

Chapter 28

Know strength, but keep to gentleness.

Know brightness, but stay close to humility.

Know honor, but do not leave simplicity.

Then you remain a channel of deep power.

What is whole does not need constant display.

When carved up by ambition,

life loses its natural force.

The wise return to the uncarved state:

useful, plain, and inwardly complete.

Chapter 29

Those who try to seize the world

and improve it by force will fail.

The world is a living reality,

not a machine for private will.

Some things move ahead.

Some follow behind.

Some breathe softly.

Some strain.

Some grow strong.

Some weaken.

The wise do not push life past its nature.

They avoid excess, aggression, and overreach.

Chapter 30

One who serves with the Way

does not dominate through violence.

Force easily returns to the one who uses it.

Where armies settle, hardship follows.

After triumph, famine and bitterness remain.

Do what is necessary.

Do not glorify power.

Complete the task without pride.

Complete it without possession.

Complete it without triumphalism.

What grows beyond its proper measure

already begins to decline.

Chapter 31

Weapons are instruments of fear.

Even when necessary,

they are not objects of celebration.

The wise person uses them reluctantly.

Peace is preferred.

Victory is not a festival,

for victory means that suffering has been spread.

To delight in conquest is to delight in harm.

Therefore even success in conflict

should be marked with sorrow and restraint.

Chapter 32

The Way is forever simple and uncarved.

Though hidden and seemingly small,

nothing can command it.

If leaders could remain true to it,

life would settle by itself.

When naming and dividing begin,

complications multiply.

Names are useful,

but they should not replace reality.

Know when to stop.

The Way in the world is like streams

returning to the sea.

Chapter 33

To understand others is intelligence.

To understand yourself is wisdom.

To conquer others requires force.

To master yourself requires strength.

To know you have enough is richness.

To stay with your path is endurance.

To die without being forgotten

by what you have lived

is lasting presence.

Chapter 34

The great Way flows everywhere.

It nourishes all things

and does not refuse them.

It completes its work

and does not claim credit.

It clothes and feeds life without ruling it.

Because it does not call itself great,

its greatness is real.

The wise learn from this.

They do not inflate themselves.

Therefore what they do becomes substantial.

Chapter 35

Hold to the central vision

and people can feel safe in your presence.

Offer them frenzy and they soon grow tired.

Offer them shallow excitement and it quickly fades.

The Way is quiet and does not seduce the senses.

Looked at, it is not dazzling.

Listened to, it is not dramatic.

Used, it never runs out.

Chapter 36

What is to be shrunk

must first be allowed to expand.

What is to be weakened may first appear strong.

What is to be cast down often rises first.

What is to be taken may first be given.

This is the subtle logic of reversal.

The soft can outlast the hard.

The hidden can overcome the obvious.

Therefore the wise do not flaunt

sharp tools before the crowd.

Chapter 37

The Way does nothing

in the sense of forcing nothing,

yet nothing is left undone.

If leaders could live from this,

people would transform themselves.

If restless desire arose,

simplicity would quiet it.

When there is little private grasping,

life becomes easier to govern.

Stillness is not passivity.

It is action free from needless interference.

Chapter 38

High virtue does not keep checking

whether it is virtuous.

That is why it is virtue.

Lower virtue tries to preserve

an image of goodness.

That is why it strains.

The highest goodness acts without calculation.

Lower goodness acts with self-conscious purpose.

When the Way is lost, virtue is discussed.

When virtue is lost, morality is imposed.

When morality is lost, ritual hardens.

Ritual is the thin shell left behind

when living truth fades.

Chapter 39

Those who are whole are whole

because they live from wholeness.

Sky is clear through wholeness.

Earth is steady through wholeness.

Spirit is alive through wholeness.

Valleys are full through wholeness.

Creatures flourish through wholeness.

Leaders are secure when they do not

separate themselves from the source.

Lose that unity and fragmentation begins.

Chapter 40

Return is the movement of the Way.

Yielding is the method of the Way.

Everything visible arises from being.

Being itself arises

from what no thing can possess.

So when life seems to move backward,

look again.

Return is not failure.

It is the path

by which what is true

renews itself.

Chapter 41

When the wise hear the Way, they practice it.

When the half-committed hear it, they waver.

When the shallow hear it, they laugh.

If they did not laugh, it would not be the Way.

The Way appears plain and therefore is overlooked.

It seems to lower what pride wants to raise.

It seems to empty what vanity wants to fill.

Great truth is often hidden by simplicity.

Chapter 42

The Way gives rise to unity.

Unity gives rise to polarity.

Polarity gives rise to relationship.

Relationship gives rise

to the many forms of life.

Everything carries complementary forces

and seeks harmony.

Too much isolation damages.

Too much aggression breaks balance.

What people hate to be called—

small, low, dependent—

often names the condition

in which strength quietly grows.

Chapter 43

What is most soft can enter what is most hard.

What has no fixed form can move

where there is no opening.

This shows the power of non-force.

Teaching without domination.

Influence without pressure.

Effectiveness without noise.

Few understand how much can be done

by what does not insist.

Chapter 44

Which matters more:

your name or your life.

Which matters more:

your possessions or your peace.

Which hurts more:

gaining at the cost of yourself,

or losing what was never stable.

Excessive attachment

always creates hidden loss.

Knowing when enough is enough,

is to know enough.

Knowing when to stop prevents danger.

This is how one endures.

Chapter 45

What is most complete may appear incomplete,

yet its use does not fail.

What is most full may appear empty,

yet it cannot be exhausted.

What is most straight may seem crooked.

What is most skilled may appear clumsy.

What is most eloquent may speak simply.

Restless movement can defeat cold.

Stillness can defeat heat.

Clarity grows from inner balance.

Chapter 46

When the Way is present,

even strong horses are used

for ordinary work.

When the Way is absent,

breeding for war becomes admirable.

No misfortune is greater

than not knowing contentment.

No fault is greater than endless wanting.

One who knows enough is rich.

One who can stop is safe.

Desire without measure

turns order into conflict.

Chapter 47

You do not need to travel everywhere

to understand the pattern of life.

The farther you chase after certainty,

the less you may really see.

The wise person knows by being present.

They discern by watching what is near.

They accomplish without frantic movement.

Depth is not gained

by mere accumulation of impressions.

Chapter 48

In the pursuit of knowledge,

something is added every day.

In the pursuit of the Way,

something is let go every day.

Less forcing.

Less clutter.

Less self-assertion.

Until action becomes so aligned

that it no longer feels like strain.

When nothing is forced, much can be done.

The world is won by those

who do not try to grab it.

Chapter 49

The wise person does not have a rigid private mind.

They meet people where they are.

They are good to the good.

They are also good to the difficult,

because goodness is their way of being.

They trust the trustworthy.

They also give trust space to grow

in the untrustworthy,

because trust is their way of meeting life.

Thus they become a steady heart

among many hearts.

Chapter 50

People move between birth and death

without understanding how to live.

Some pursue life in ways that waste it.

Some pursue safety in ways

that increases danger.

Why?

Because they do not know how to

inhabit the present without excess.

One who lives simply and fully

does not create so many openings for harm.

This does not make them immortal.

It makes them less divided against life.

Chapter 51

The Way gives life.

Virtue nurtures it.

Circumstances shape it.

Experience completes it.

Therefore all things honor the Way

and value virtue,

not because they are commanded to,

but because life is sustained by them.

To give life, to guide growth,

to help without possessing,

to lead without controlling:

this is profound integrity.

Chapter 52

The world has a source.

Knowing the source, we understand the children.

Knowing the children, we can return to the source.

Close the doors of endless craving.

Guard the openings

through which confusion enters.

Then life can remain steady.

If you spend yourself without measure,

you become difficult to recover.

What is small should be seen while it is still small.

That is clarity.

Chapter 53

If I had even a little understanding,

I would walk the great Way

and only fear straying from it.

The great Way is smooth,

yet people love side paths of display,

profit, and excess.

When palaces shine while fields are neglected,

something is out of order.

When luxury grows beside hunger,

something is out of order.

This is not the Way.

It is pride living off imbalance.

Chapter 54

What is well rooted cannot be easily uprooted.

What is well held cannot be easily lost.

Cultivate integrity in yourself and it becomes real.

Cultivate it in the family and it grows.

Cultivate it in the community and it spreads.

Cultivate it in the country and it shapes

institutions.

Cultivate it in the world and it becomes a pattern.

How do we know this.

By watching how inner life becomes outer life.

Chapter 55

One who is deeply aligned with life is like a

newborn child.

Soft, yet vigorous.

Open, yet whole.

Without fixed strategy, yet close to original power.

Harmony gathers naturally where there is little

inner division.

Too much strain ages the spirit before its time.

When vitality is forced, it burns out.

What is fully alive does not need to prove that it is

alive.

Chapter 56

Those who know deeply do not rush to speak.

Those who speak endlessly have not yet settled.

Close the mouth when words are only agitation.

Guard the senses from excess.

Soften sharpness.

Untie knots.

Lower glare.

Learn to move among the world

without becoming trapped

by praise or blame.

This is called profound sameness.

Chapter 57

Govern with straightforward means.

Meet conflict with restraint.

Win a people not by overregulation

but by not exhausting them.

The more prohibitions increase,

the poorer life often becomes.

The more sharp instruments multiply,

the more disorder grows.

The more clever schemes spread,

the more strange results appear.

So the wise ruler says:

I do not overact,

and people become balanced.

Chapter 58

When rule is gentle,

people remain simple and honest.

When rule is harsh,

people become guarded and cunning.

Misfortune leans on fortune.

Fortune hides in misfortune.

Who can draw the final line between them.

The wise person does not become rigid.

They are firm without cutting.

Clear without dazzling.

Straight without pressing.

Because life changes,

wisdom avoids extremity.

Chapter 59

In governing others

and in caring for your own life,

nothing is better than moderation.

Moderation means returning early

before excess takes hold.

Returning early means storing strength.

Stored strength makes resilience possible.

Resilience makes long stewardship possible.

A deep root and a firm base:

this is the way of lasting vision.

Chapter 60

Governing a large country

is like cooking a small fish.

Too much handling ruins it.

Where the Way is present,

disruptive forces lose their grip.

Not because power has crushed them,

but because no one is feeding chaos.

When ruler and people stop injuring one another,

virtue gathers itself.

Chapter 61

A great country

should be like a low basin

into which rivers flow.

What is low receives.

What receives can unite.

The receptive often overcomes

the assertive,

not by attack,

but by making room.

If the large can place itself below the small,

and the small can trust what is large,

both benefit.

Power becomes legitimate

when it is willing to stoop.

Chapter 62

The Way is the hidden support of all things.

It is a treasure to the good

and a refuge for those not yet good.

Fine words may win respect.

Fine deeds may win advantage.

But the Way does not reject anyone.

Why did the ancients value it.

Because through it one can find what was sought

and be forgiven for what was misplaced.

Chapter 63

Act before complications multiply.

Set things in order while they are still manageable.

A giant tree grows from a small shoot.

A tower rises from a heap of earth.

A long journey begins under the foot.

Those who rush to seize completion often spoil it.

Those who cling to the end lose the process.

The wise stay attentive to the small beginning.

Chapter 64

What is at rest is easy to hold.

What has not yet appeared is easy to prevent.

What is fragile is easy to break.

What is subtle is easy to disperse.

Deal with things before they become difficult.

Order things before they become chaotic.

The wise do not force grand endings.

They attend to early signs

and avoid unnecessary damage.

Chapter 65

The ancient guides

did not try to dazzle people with complexity.

They helped them return to simplicity.

When there is too much clever manipulation,

life becomes hard to govern.

Using cunning to manage

a people harms both ruler and ruled.

Living from simplicity blesses both.

To know this pattern is called deep virtue.

Deep virtue is not narrow.

It moves opposite to ambition

and returns life to balance.

Chapter 66

Rivers and seas become kings of valleys because

they stay below them.

That is why all streams flow toward them.

If you want to lead people, speak from below them.

If you want to guide them, do not stand over them.

Then leadership does not feel like oppression.

Because the wise do not contend for position,

people do not feel pushed aside by them.

Chapter 67

I have three things I value and keep.

The first is compassion.

The second is moderation.

The third is not placing myself above others.

With compassion, one can be courageous.

With moderation, one can be generous.

With humility, one can lead.

When courage is pursued without compassion,

it becomes brutality.

When ambition outruns humility,

leadership collapses.

Chapter 68

A good warrior is not warlike.

A good fighter is not driven by rage.

A good conqueror does not relish domination.

A good leader serves those they lead.

This is called the virtue of not contending.

It is the ability to use human strength

without feeding human aggression.

It is also the old lesson:

to work with others, leave room for them.

Chapter 69

In conflict, it is wiser to receive

than to charge blindly.

Better to take a step back

than to advance without measure.

To fight without hatred,

to defend without arrogance,

to engage without underestimating the other:

this is real skill.

There is no greater mistake

than making light of resistance.

When struggle cannot be avoided,

the one who stays inwardly sober

is nearest to winning.

Chapter 70

My words are easy to understand

and easy to practice,

yet few understand them

and few practice them.

Why.

Because people seek complexity

and neglect what is plain.

Words have a source.

Actions have a root.

When that root is not known,

life becomes confused.

The wise wear rough cloth

and carry jade within:

outwardly simple, inwardly rich.

Chapter 71

To know that you do not fully know is health.

To imagine that you already know is sickness.

Once you become aware of this sickness,

healing begins.

The wise are not trapped

by false certainty

because they see the danger of it.

Clear seeing starts

with intellectual humility.

Chapter 72

When people no longer fear power,

greater disorder approaches.

Do *not press people until they cannot breathe.*

Do *not narrow their lives until resentment hardens.*

The *wise know themselves*

but do not display themselves.

They *respect themselves*

but do not inflate themselves.

They *let go of vanity*

and choose what preserves dignity.

Chapter 73

Boldness in reckless daring leads toward death.

Boldness in careful restraint leads toward life.

Both are called courage,

but they are not the same.

Who knows why heaven seems to favor one

and not the other.

The Way of heaven does not struggle,

yet it knows how to prevail.

It does not speak,

yet it knows how to answer.

Chapter 74

If people are not afraid of death,

threats of death cannot control them.

If a ruler constantly tries to take the place

of the great forces of life and death,

that ruler wounds the order they rely on.

There is a master carpenter who cuts.

To seize the axe in their place

is to risk cutting your own hand.

Power should respect limits.

Chapter 75

People become hungry

when those above them consume too much.

People become difficult to govern

when their lives are overmanaged.

People take life lightly

when living has become too hard.

Therefore one who does not cling

anxiously to mere survival

can actually value life more deeply.

Oppression makes people desperate.

Simplicity makes room for sanity.

Chapter 76

At birth, living things are soft and flexible.

At death, they are rigid and dry.

Hardness belongs to what is nearing its end.

Softness belongs to what is alive.

Thus a rigid army does not win for long.

A hard tree is soon cut down.

The strong and stiff are placed below.

The soft and yielding rise.

Chapter 77

The Way of heaven is like drawing a bow:

what is high is lowered,

what is low is raised,

what is excessive is reduced,

what is lacking is supplied.

Human ambition often does the opposite.

It takes from what lacks

and gives to what already has.

The wise person has enough and keeps giving.

They act without hoarding the credit.

Chapter 78

Nothing in the world is softer than water,

yet nothing can better wear down what is hard.

The weak overcomes the strong.

The yielding overcomes the rigid.

Everyone knows this,

yet few can live it.

To bear what others reject

is often the beginning of real strength.

Chapter 79

After a deep conflict, some resentment remains.

So how can one insist on perfect settlement.

The wise do not press

their advantage to the last point.

They keep to their side of the agreement

without demanding humiliation from the other.

The Way of heaven has no favorites,

but it stays with those

who do not abandon what is fair.

Chapter 80

Let there be a small community

with simple means.

Let tools exist

without becoming a cause of restless ambition.

Let people take life seriously enough

not to chase unnecessary danger.

Let them enjoy their food,

value their homes, and love their ordinary ways.

Even if nearby places are close enough to hear,

there is no need to rush everywhere.

A good life does not require constant expansion.

Chapter 81

True words are not usually decorated.

Decorated words are not always true.

The good do not need to argue.

Those who are always arguing

are seldom at peace.

Those who truly know

are not obsessed with appearing learned.

The wise do not hoard.

The more they help others, the richer life becomes.

The Way of heaven benefits and does not injure.

The way of the wise is to serve without competing.

Further Reading and Scientific References

The Storytelling Monkey: Where Neuroscience ends and Wisdom begins – Steve Brandl (2026)

The Storytelling Monkey and the Web of Life – Steve Brandl (2026)

Anatomy Trains: Myofascial Meridians for Manual Therapists and Movement Professionals, 4th Edition – Thomas W. Myers

Fascial Manipulation Practical Part – First Level, Second Level, and Third Level – Luigi Stecco, Carla Stecco, Antonio Stecco

Fascial Manipulation for Internal Dysfunction Practical Part – Luigi Stecco, Antonio Stecco

Functional Atlas of the Human Fascial System – Carla Stecco

Fascia in Sport and Movement, 2nd Edition – Robert Schleip, Jan Wilke

The Spark in the Machine: How the Science of Acupuncture Explains the Mysteries of Western Medicine – Daniel Keown

Fascial Fitness – Robert Schleip, Johanna Bayer

Breath: The New Science of a Lost Art – James Nestor

The Body Keeps the Score – Bessel van der Kolk

Being You: A New Science of Consciousness – Anil Seth

The Hidden Spring – Mark Solms

A current search for fascia on PubMed Central reveals over 90,000 publications. Select pivotal research papers include:

Evidence of connective tissue involvement in acupuncture – Helene M. Langevin et al.

Role of fasciae in nonspecific low back pain – Gulia Casato, Carla Stecco, Riccardo Busin

Effectiveness of trigger point dry needling for multiple body regions – Robert Boyles et al.

Fascia Mobility, Proprioception, and Myofascial Pain – Helene M. Langevin

Painful connections: densification versus fibrosis of fascia – Piero G. Pavan et al.

Hyaluronan within fascia in the etiology of myofascial pain – Carla Stecco et al.

Deep fascia as a potential source of pain – Kobi Weiss, Leonid Kalichman

Cellular Reorganization Plays a Vital Role in Acupuncture Analgesia – Conner E. Liddle, Richard E. Harris

Connective Tissue Fibroblast Response to Acupuncture – Helene M. Langevin et al.

The strain-generated electrical potential in cartilaginous tissues – Philip Poillot et al.

Dry needling: a literature review with implications for clinical practice guidelines – James Dunning et al.

Fascial Disorders: Implications for Treatment – Antonio Stecco et al.

Evidence of a new hidden neural network into deep fasciae – Caterina Fede et al.

Meaning of the Solid and Liquid Fascia to Reconsider the Model of Biotensegrity – Bruno Bordoni et al.

Relationship of acupuncture points and meridians to connective tissue planes – Helene M. Langevin, Jason A. Yandow

The deep fascia and its role in chronic pain and pathological conditions – Flemming Kondrup et al.

Acupuncture, connective tissue, and peripheral sensory modulation – Helene M. Langevin

An in vitro assay of collagen fiber alignment by acupuncture needle rotation – Margaret Julias et al.

Effectiveness of Manual and Electrical Acupuncture for Chronic Non-specific Low Back Pain – Josielli Comachio et al.

Table of Contents

www.ingramcontent.com/pod-product-compliance
Lightning Source LLC
LaVergne TN
LVHW090306210926
848480LV00001B/153

* 9 7 9 8 2 3 3 0 6 9 0 9 3 *